THE DOC C
GUIDE TO HEALING HERBS

In this essential guide you can discover the amazing power of easy-to-find herbs to help ease common conditions, including:

- acne
- hangover
- heartburn
- asthma
- high blood pressure
- headache
- coughs

- anemia
- dermatitis
- hepatitis
- high cholesterol
- boils
- bad breath
- cold sores
- bronchitis

- ear infections
- fever
- bruising
- common colds
- indigestion
- blood clots

and more . . .

Don't miss THE DOCTOR'S COMPLETE GUIDE TO HEALING FOODS, a Berkley paperback available at bookstores everywhere.

THE DOCTOR'S COMPLETE GUIDE TO HEALING HERBS

David Kessler, M.D.,
with Sheila Buff

Produced by The Philip Lief Group, Inc.

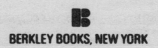

BERKLEY BOOKS, NEW YORK

NOTE: Medical research about the healing properties of different hebs is ongoing and subject to interpretation. Although every effort has been made to include the most up-to-date information in this book, there can be no guarantee that what we know about these herbs will not change with time. The reader should bear in mind that this book should not be used for self-diagnosis or self-treatment; he or she should consult appropriate medical professionals regarding all medical problems and before undertaking any major dietary changes or taking any vitamin or dietary supplements.

THE DOCTOR'S COMPLETE GUIDE TO HEALING HERBS

A Berkley Book / published by arrangement with
The Philip Lief Group, Inc.

PRINTING HISTORY
Berkley edition / June 1996

All rights reserved.
Copyright © 1996 by The Philip Lief Group, Inc.
Produced by The Philip Lief Group, Inc.
This book may not be reproduced in whole or in part,
by mimeograph or any other means, without permission.
For information address:
The Philip Lief Group, Inc., 130 Wall Street, Princeton, New Jersey 08540.

The Putnam Berkley World Wide Web site address is
http://www.berkley.com

ISBN: 0-425-15342-8

BERKLEY®
Berkley Books are published by
The Berkley Publishing Group, a member of Penguin Putnam Inc.,
200 Madison Avenue, New York, New York 10016.
BERKLEY and the "B" design are trademarks
belonging to Berkley Publishing Corporation.

PRINTED IN THE UNITED STATES OF AMERICA

10   9   8   7   6   5   4

❖ Contents

❖ Introduction

Herbs and Your Health

The explosion of interest in herbal healing today reflects a growing desire among many people to take personal responsibility for their own well-being. As a physician, I encourage my patients to be actively involved in their own health care. I believe that many minor medical problems can be safely and effectively treated with simple herbal remedies. I also believe that herbs and diet can play an important supportive role in the management of many serious health problems. But as a responsible health professional, I can't recommend an herbal remedy simply because some people claim it works or because a preliminary study hints that it might be helpful. Herbs are not magic; they will not miraculously cure cancer or arthritis or even the common cold. Herbs should have more of a place in today's medicine, but in most cases, they should not substitute for standard medical treatment.

Many of the claims made for particular herbs or herb mixtures are exaggerated or based on fractured science. If an herb is worthless, unproven, or harmful, I say so. When it comes to herbs, my patients deserve honest information based on reliable evidence. In this book, I have tried to present the most recent developments in herbal medicine in a fair and truthful way.

Herbal Cautions

Herbs are generally safe for the self-treatment of minor ailments in healthy adults. However, herbs and other natural remedies are not a substitute for professional medical care. If you wish to use herbs in medicinal amounts, first discuss doing so with your doctor. Do not combine any medicines, even nonprescription drugs, with herbs. If you have any sort of chronic condition such as asthma, diabetes, heart disease, high blood pressure, or a clotting disorder, discuss herbal remedies with your doctor before trying them.

Don't give medicinal doses of herbs to children under age two. People in poor health or over age sixty-five should use herbal remedies cautiously, starting with small doses and gradually increasing them. Sometimes the recommended adult dosage of an herb may cause discomfort or side effects. If this happens to you, take less of the herb or stop using it altogether.

Most importantly, if the symptoms for which you are using the herb don't go away or significantly improve within a week to ten days, *see your doctor.* You could have a serious medical problem.

What Is an Herb?

Technically speaking, an herb is a perennial or annual plant with a fleshy stem. As the word is more generally used in this book and elsewhere, an herb is any plant with a medicinal or culinary use. In this larger sense of the word, then, herbs can be the seeds, leaves, stems, flowers, roots, berries, or even barks of plants that are used for healing. Some herbs, such as black pepper, are used primarily as spices; others, such as ginger, have dual uses as seasonings and as medicines. Most of the herbs discussed here, however, are known chiefly for their real or imagined healing value.

A Brief History of Herbal Medicine

Herbs of various sorts have been used for healing for millennia. Ancient Egyptian documents more than four thousand years old record herbal remedies. Traditional Chinese herbal medicine is at least that old, and the Ayurvedic herbal medicine of India dates back equally far. The European herbal tradition began when the ancient Greek physician Hippocrates, the father of medicine, recorded numerous herbal prescriptions and their uses over two thousand years ago. By the beginning of the third century A.D., the Roman physician Galen had standardized many herbal formulas. European medicine remained heavily reliant on the works of Galen for centuries to come, with additional knowledge from the Islamic world gradually creeping into the herbal books. Even so, herbal medicine became largely a collection of blindly obeyed ancient dictums, folklore, and superstitions. By the 1500s, the great Swiss physician Paracelsus had begun to apply some logic to the art of medicine. He rejected Galen's theory of humors and instead advocated the use of specific remedies for specific illnesses. He was probably the first Western physician to use opium as a painkiller. Paracelsus, however, was also an alchemist. In addition to his belief that lead could be somehow transmuted to gold (he never succeeded), he also believed herbs that happened to resemble a part of the body or a symptom could be used to treat related diseases. In the Doctrine of Signatures, as this belief came to be called, dandelion flowers were considered a good treatment for jaundice, because the yellow flowers resemble the yellow color of the patient's skin. Perhaps because of a lucky coincidence or two, the Doctrine of Signatures caught on—and remains with us. For example, the herb eyebright, whose leaves resemble bloodshot eyes, is to this day recommended by some herbalists as an eyewash, even though it is completely ineffective and potentially dangerous.

At the same time, Paracelsus did inspire his followers to systematically survey the herbs around them. This work led to the great age of herbals in the seventeenth century, during which beautiful books by Gerard, Parkinson, Culpepper, and others described and illustrated medicinal herbs. With many wildly inaccurate descriptions and vague or fanciful recommendations, the beneficial results were often nonexistent. Inexplicably, these historical documents continue to be used as serious references by some herbalists.

As Western medicine became more systematic, scientific, academic, and hierarchial, traditional herbal medicine was gradually discredited and only kept alive by folklore and the hands of local healers. Given some of the harsh and worthless orthodox medical treatments that prevailed until as late as the start of the twentieth century, it's not surprising that a countervailing school of herbal medicine arose in the United States in the 1830s. Known as Eclecticism, this system was a form of scientific herbalism that used an orthodox medical approach to diagnosis but treated illness with botanical remedies, including those drawn from Native American lore. Eclecticism remained quite popular for decades, but by the beginning of the twentieth century, the movement had lost scientific and academic support. Eclectic physicians faded from the medical scene.

At the same time, advances in chemistry made it possible for the organic compounds found in many plants to be synthesized in the laboratory. Purified, concentrated drugs in measured doses replaced medicinal herbs. Overall, this more systematic approach to pharmacology was a great boon to patients, because it led to easier and more accurate dosing. As herbs became less and less a part of mainstream medicine, the pharmacists who knew their uses had little call for their knowledge. By the 1930s, standard medical and pharmaceutical reference books such as *The United States Pharmacopeia* and *The National Formulary* started removing herbs of unproven effectiveness from their listings. Today, these volumes offer information on few herbs, so some herbalists refer back to editions that are decades out of date.

Herbs and Government Regulation

Fraudulent, often dangerous medicines that made extravagant claims for miraculous cures were one of the targets of the Food and Drugs Act of 1906, which among other things created the federal Food and Drug Administration. The 1906 act prohibited adulterated drugs and effectively eliminated many of the worthless patent and herbal medicines that were in widespread use during the late nineteenth century. Laws regulating the safety and effectiveness of herbal medicines didn't come about until 1938, with the passage of the Food, Drug, and Cosmetic Act, which stated that any substance sold as a drug must be proven safe. The 1938 act was amended in 1962 to state that drugs had to be proven not only safe but also effective. In general, these laws were of great benefit to medical consumers. They rid the shelves in pharmacies of many useless nonprescription drugs, for example, and forced the labels on other nonprescription products to be much more accurate and detailed. Among other requirements, a product could be sold as a drug for the treatment of a specific medical condition only if its active ingredients had been shown to be effective through scientific testing. Unfortunately, the labeling requirements drove most herbal remedies out of the drugstores completely. They ended up in health food stores, where they are sold as food supplements, teas, and the like. Because they are not considered drugs, the labeling on herbal remedies is not subject to the same stringencies and the ingredients are often inaccurately described. Purchasers now get their medical advice from part-time store clerks rather than trained pharmacists.

Consumers are not entirely on their own, however. The FDA maintains a list of some 250 herbs that it considers to be generally recognized as safe—the GRAS list. This, too, can be misleading, since some herbs that are on the list are not necessarily safe in medicinal doses, and herbs that are not on the list are not necessarily unsafe. The FDA does sometimes declare an herb to be unsafe, however, and that designation should be taken seriously.

Herbal Medicine Today

Thoughtful consumers have a few good sources of reliable information about herbal treatments. Much of the herbal advice given out today is still mired in folklore, hearsay, anecdote, and hype. A lot of so-called scientific evidence is based on fractured interpretations of preliminary or poorly designed studies. Ironically, consumers who are very quick to criticize orthodox medicine are just as quick to accept some of the most outrageous claims for the effectiveness of herbal remedies. Similarly, patients who are deeply suspicious of the profit motive in standard medicine often pay grossly inflated sums for worthless natural remedies. A good example is sassafras, which is marketed to bodybuilders as a natural steroid that also contains testosterone. The claims are nonsense, of course, but the sellers of these products still find willing buyers.

Fortunately, there are more and more well-trained physicians and other health care professionals who have an understanding of herbs and are willing to work with patients who want to use them. There are also many self-styled herbal practitioners, however, who lack medical knowledge and diagnostic skills. Some combine herbal medicine with untestable mystical beliefs such as astrology or numerology. Their treatments are often little more than expensive quackery. In cases of serious illness, these practitioners can do much more harm than good. If you are interested in herbal medicine, I urge you to avoid unqualified practitioners. Find an open-minded physician instead, and remain open minded yourself about the value of orthodox medical treatment.

Obtaining Herbs

Well-stocked health food stores and mail-order companies generally carry a wide range of herbs and herbal products. As discussed above, herbal products are often labeled imprecisely. For example, the common name of the herbs is usually given on the label, not the more accurate scientific binomial. The same herb can go by several different common names, however; conversely, the same common name can be applied to several different herbs.

In addition to the nomenclature problem is the problem of adulteration. Deliberately or accidentally, other herbs or inactive parts of the plant are sometimes mixed in or substituted for the desired herb. For example, the active ingredients in chamomile are mostly found in the whole flowers, but packaged chamomile often contains stems and bits of leaves. Commercial chamomile tea bags generally contain powdered or crushed flowers and stems. Chamomile oil, which is quite expensive and has a distinctive blue color, can be and often is adulterated with far cheaper synthetic blue compounds.

How and where an herb is grown, processed, and stored has a big effect on the strength of its active ingredients. Herbs should be harvested when they are mature and then dried quickly in a dark, cool place. They should be stored in glass or ceramic containers in a cool, dark place. Herbs should also be used quickly, preferably within six to twelve months from harvesting, because the volatile oils and other compounds that give herbs their value can lose their effectiveness over time. Do not use any herb that smells musty or off, is moldy, faded, or discolored, has any signs of insect infestation or obvious contamination, or seems very dry or dusty.

To be reasonably certain you are getting high-quality herbs, purchase them only from a reliable, established source. Many people like to grow or collect their own herbs. Accurately labeled seeds for most culinary herbs can be easily purchased, and these herbs usually grow well with little attention. Collecting your own herbs in the wild is another matter. Unless you have a lot of experience, you could make a serious mistake. For example, burdock root looks dangerously like the root of deadly nightshade, and confusing the two could be fatal. Wild parsley could easily be confused with poisonous water hemlock. In addition, unregulated herb gathering in the wild has actually caused some plants to become endangered. What happened to goldenseal, a popular but not very effective herb, is a good example. Because overharvesting led to restrictions on gathering this herb, it became scarce and expensive. Making matters worse, unscrupulous sellers then began to adulterate it with dried bloodroot, a powerful laxative.

Preparing Herbal Remedies

Herbs can be used in a variety of forms. The choice of form often depends on the herb itself and on the symptoms it is being used to treat. In most cases, medicinal doses are made using this standard ratio: 1 ounce (30 grams) of dried herbs or 2 ounces of fresh herbs to 2 cups (1 pint or 16 ounces or 500 milliliters) of water. An ounce by volume of most herbs is quite a bit—about a handful or approximately 5 to 7 tablespoons. The herbs will soak up about 1/2 cup of the water. Because of the quantities used, many herbal teas and other medicinal preparations have a strong taste. Try adding some honey or sugar to make the mixture more palatable.

Tea or infusion. Perhaps the simplest and most common way to use an herb is to make it into a tea or infusion. Place the herb(s) into a teapot and add boiling water. To extract the maximum benefit, cover tightly and let steep for at least fifteen minutes. Strain before drinking.

Decoction. A decoction is made by boiling the herb in water. It is generally used when the herb consists of dried roots or woody parts such as bark. Put the herbs in a saucepan and add cold water. Bring to a boil, then lower the heat and simmer gently for up to an hour or until the volume has been reduced by about a third. Strain before using.

Syrup. Many useful herbs have an unpleasant taste that can be disguised in a syrup. First prepare the herb(s) as a strong infusion or decoction. Strain the mixture into a small saucepan over low heat. Gradually stir in enough honey to make a syrup—2 tablespoons will make a thin syrup, but you can use more or less depending on your taste. Pour the mixture into a bottle and store in the refrigerator. Use within a month.

Tincture. A tincture uses alcohol instead of water to release the active ingredients from the herb. For some herbs, such as echinacea, tinctures are the most effective preparation. Many herbs are sold in tincture form using ethyl alcohol and water. To make your own, put the herb(s) into a glass or ceramic container with a tightly fitting lid. Add enough vodka to cover (do not use rubbing alcohol or wood alcohol), seal, and let stand in a cool, dark place for up to two weeks. Shake the mixture twice a day. Strain before using. Take the tincture with fruit juice to disguise the taste.

Fluid extracts. Fluid extracts are more concentrated and potent than tinctures. You can't really make them at home. Add fluid extracts to fruit juice to disguise the taste.

Capsules and tablets. Many herbs are available commercially in convenient capsule or tablet form. Capsules usually contain 200 to 250 milligrams of powdered herb(s) in a hard gelatin casing. Tablets usually combine powdered herbs with cornstarch, milk sugar, or some other neutral base; tablets vary in their dosage. You can make capsules by purchasing empty cases at the health food store and filling them yourself.

Herbal oils. Commercial herbal oils are made using a distillation process that is far too complex and expensive to do at home. Instead, you can make a less-concentrated oil by placing 2 ounces of dried herb (4 ounces of fresh herb) in a glass container. Add 2 cups olive oil, canola oil, or safflower oil; cover; and let stand in a warm, dark place for three to five days. Strain into another container and store in a dark place. Alternatively, combine the herbs and oil in a saucepan and heat gently for one hour. Do not let the mixture boil. Let cool, then strain into another container.

Creams and ointments. Creams and ointments are useful for treating minor skin problems. To make them, first prepare an herbal oil as described above. Melt 1 to 2 ounces of beeswax in a double boiler and stir in the herbal oil. The more beeswax you use, the firmer the mixture will be.

Compresses, poultices, and plasters. Sometimes the best way to use an herb is externally. Compresses and poultices are especially useful for skin problems and soreness in muscles or joints. To make a compress, soak a small towel or washcloth in hot (not more than 180°F) herbal tea. Wring it out and place it on the affected area; cover with a dry towel to keep the heat in. Leave the compress in place for several minutes. When it cools, remove it and replace it with a fresh one. Repeat several times for up to thirty minutes. Stop using the compress if it causes discomfort or the area becomes very red.

To make a poultice, begin by making a tea from dried herbs. Then, strain off the liquid and place the warm herbs directly against the skin at the affected area. Hold the herbs in place with a towel. Because the herbs are in direct contact with the skin, use only mild, nonirritating herbs such as slippery elm or burdock in poultices. Stop using the poultice if it causes discomfort or the area becomes very red.

Generally, plasters are made using strong herbs, such as cayenne or mustard. To make a plaster, combine the powdered herb with water and, if necessary, enough flour, oatmeal, or cornstarch to form a thin paste. Spread the paste on a piece of cheesecloth and fold the cloth so that the paste is covered by several layers. Place the plaster on the affected area and leave it there until it becomes uncomfortably warm on the skin. Do not leave the plaster in place for more than ten minutes or skin blistering may occur. Do not use plasters on babies, children, the elderly, or anyone with very sensitive skin.

Herbal Dosages

How much of an herbal remedy should you take? How often should you take it? If you are a healthy adult, you can follow these general rules of thumb: For teas and decoctions, take 1/2 cup three times a day. Tinctures and fluid extracts are far more potent and require much smaller doses. In general, use between 5 drops and 1 tablespoon three times a day, but read the label for directions. If you use a syrup, take 1 to 2 tablespoons three times a day. For most herbs in capsule form, the dose is 2 or 3 capsules taken two or three times daily. Herbs in tablet form vary in their potency; read the label.

The best dosage for you may be more or less than the amounts suggested above, and some cautious experimentation may be needed to find the dose that works well for you. Start with the basic amount and adjust the dosage in small increments until it meets your needs. If one basic dose causes discomfort or side effects, take less of the herb, take it less often, or stop using it completely. If your symptoms get worse within a few days, if they remain the same, or fail to get noticeably better within a week to ten days, *see your doctor.*

Ailments and Conditions

❖ Acne

Unsightly, annoying acne blemishes occur when the oil ducts in the skin of your face (and sometimes chest and back) get plugged up. The trapped oil (sebum) forms a whitehead. The duct eventually ruptures, resulting in irritation and inflammation—in other words, pimples. Acne can be caused or aggravated by cosmetics, high humidity, sweating, skin irritation or friction, and some prescription drugs.

Hormones play a major role in plugged oil ducts. Both boys and girls begin to produce more of a hormone called androgen as they enter puberty. This hormone stimulates the oil ducts, causing them to grow larger and start producing oil. The process often goes haywire, especially if there is a family tendency toward acne, and excess oil plugs the ducts. Many adult women continue to be plagued by acne flare-ups that coincide with hormonal fluctuations brought about by their menstrual cycles. Stress also increases hormone production, which worsens acne.

Despite many popular myths, there is little clear connection between diet and acne. There is no evidence, for example, that chocolate, soft drinks, greasy foods, or dairy products cause acne. However, some evidence suggests that food high in iodine may cause acne flareups. Seaweed, including kelp, wakame, and nori, is very high in iodine. If you notice a connection between eating those foods and in-

13

creased pimples, you might be sensitive to iodine. Try eliminating seaweed and iodine-rich foods from your diet. Furthermore, many herbalists recommend a diet low in fat and
junk food and high in fresh fruits and vegetables. A cup of
red clover or raspberry leaf tea daily is also recommended.

The first step in controlling acne is good hygiene to remove excess sebum. Wash your face gently with pure soap
and warm water, and then pat your skin dry with a towel.
Scrubbing hard while washing or drying may actually make
your acne worse. Choose an ordinary soap without moisturizers or fragrances. Ordinary soaps are as effective as medicated facial soaps, since the active ingredients in medicated
soaps are just rinsed away. Abrasive cleaners can sometimes
help unclog pores. Organic formulations usually contain
ground-up almond or walnut shells. Never rub these products vigorously into the skin. Apply in a circular motion
using very little pressure. Be careful not to get these products in your eyes. If you do, rinse your eyes thoroughly with
clean water.

Herbal steam facials help open your pores, loosen dead
skin cells and deep dirt, and kill germs on the skin that can
worsen your acne. Adding herbs to the water can make the
facial more effective and enjoyable. Overall, lavender is an
effective germ-killer and has a delicate, pleasant aroma. Red
clover is another herb useful for acne. For oily skin, try
adding equal parts licorice root, lemongrass, and rose petals.
If your skin has both oily and dry areas, try using a mixture
of equal parts lavender, peppermint, and chamomile flowers. Let the steam soften and cleanse your skin for a few
minutes, rinse with cool water to close the pores, and pat dry
gently with a towel. Repeat the facial treatment three times a
week.

Many skin doctors recommend applying benzoyl peroxide, a very effective nonprescription treatment for acne, to
the skin. It helps open clogged pores and dries lesions. It
may also help kill bacteria that can lead to infection. Tea tree
oil is an effective herbal alternative to benzoyl peroxide, although the positive results may take a little longer to
achieve. Apply the oil to the affected area several times a

day. If skin irritation more severe than mild drying and chapping occurs, try using a less concentrated form or applying it less often. If skin irritation, swelling, or redness persists, however, stop using tea tree oil. Avoid putting the oil around your mouth, eyes, and nostrils.

Try applying calendula cream or ointment to individual blemishes. Arnica tincture or cream applied to the blemishes may be helpful, but can sometimes cause redness or irritation. Stop using it if this occurs. Aloe vera gel is another herbal remedy that can be applied directly to the blemishes. You could also try making a lotion from equal parts pureed fresh cabbage leaves and witch hazel.

❖ Age Spots

Age spots, sometimes called liver spots, are flat, irregular brownish blotches that appear on your skin, particularly the backs of your hands, as you get older. Unsightly but basically harmless, age spots are caused by excess sun exposure. To avoid worsening the problem, stay out of the sun. The name liver spots is a little misleading; the spots are only very rarely the result of a poorly functioning liver.

Some herbalists claim that poultices of ginseng, gotu kola, licorice, or sarsaparilla can help fade age spots. On the other hand, some herbs could actually contribute to the formation of age spots. Psoralen, a substance found in parsley, citrus rinds, and parsnips, can make your skin more sensitive to sunlight. If you go out into the sun after handling these foods, your hands may sunburn more easily, making them more susceptible to age spots later on. Bergamot oil, a substance often found in perfume, skin creams, and other beauty products, can have a similar effect.

If the blotches are reddish brown or purplish, they may be caused by a condition called senile purpura. Because the skin has become less elastic with age, the tiny blood vessels under the surface are damaged. Blood may seep out of the vessels and collect in blotches under the skin. The spots gradually fade away, but they are likely to recur. In almost all cases, the spots are harmless, but you should see a physician if you notice them.

It's possible to mistake skin cancer lesions for age spots. If your age spots change shape or color, bleed, become raised, or take on a pearly color, see your doctor immediately.

❖ AIDS

The human immunodeficiency virus (HIV) causes acquired immunodeficiency syndrome (AIDS), an incurable illness that weakens the body's ability to fight off infections from bacteria, viruses, and parasites. HIV can be passed from person to person only through body fluids such as blood, semen, and vaginal fluid. Most people infected with AIDS in the United States today caught it by having unprotected anal, vaginal, or oral sex with an infected person, or by injecting drugs using needles and syringes shared with an infected person. Babies born to HIV-positive women often develop AIDS in early childhood. Homosexual men and intravenous drug users statistically run the highest risk of getting AIDS, although growing numbers of heterosexual women and men are contracting the disease.

Since 1981, when it was first formally recognized, over 400,000 people have been diagnosed with AIDS; of that total, nearly 250,000 have died. Currently, about 1 million people in the U.S. are infected with HIV.

Because HIV can't live for very long outside the body, it can't be passed easily from one person to the next. You can't get AIDS from touching or being around infected people, although precautions must be taken to avoid contact with their blood and body fluids. Since 1985, all donated blood has been carefully screened for HIV infection. Today, you are very unlikely to contract AIDS from a blood transfusion or from a blood-based product.

With some rare exceptions, everyone infected with HIV will eventually develop AIDS, although people infected with HIV may remain in good health for a long time—eight to eleven years or possibly even longer. People who know they are HIV-positive need to carefully guard their health by eating a low-fat, high-fiber diet that provides at least 100 percent of recommended daily vitamin and mineral requirements. Most doctors also advise HIV patients to get plenty of rest, avoid stress, and stop smoking and drinking alcohol. Garlic, a natural antibiotic, may be taken as a supplement to help ward off infections. Some HIV patients feel that taking odorless garlic capsules every day helps them avoid minor illnesses. Another antibacterial herb that some HIV patients find helpful is echinacea.

The early symptoms of the onset of AIDS include recurrent fever, night sweats, constant fatigue, diarrhea, appetite loss, rapid weight loss, and swollen lymph glands. In the later stages of AIDS, patients are extremely susceptible to opportunistic infections that their weakened immune systems can't fight off. Illnesses such as thrush, pneumonia, and a type of skin cancer called Kaposi's sarcoma are common. The powerful antiviral drug AZT along with more effective treatment of secondary illnesses such as pneumocystis carinii pneumonia may help improve the quality of life for AIDS patients and prolong their healthy periods.

Sadly, there is no cure for AIDS. There is also no evidence that any food can actually kill HIV or prevent the development of AIDS symptoms. Megadoses of vitamins and nutrients haven't proven effective, either. In fact, in some cases they may be harmful. Megadoses of vitamin C, for example can cause diarrhea, which could be harmful or even fatal to an AIDS patient. However, many doctors do advise supplemental doses of magnesium, selenium, and zinc, since the levels of these minerals are often found to be low in AIDS patients. Dandelion is a good source of zinc, magnesium, niacin, and many B vitamins, including vitamin B_{12}; gotu kola has magnesium; kelp has selenium and zinc; and garlic contains selenium, zinc, and magnesium. Alfalfa, which is often recommended by naturopaths to detoxify the liver, is an excellent all-around source of vitamins, minerals, and other nutrients. Alfalfa can be taken in capsule or liquid form or eaten as sprouts. Some HIV and AIDS patients claim to find red clover flowers, which are high in all the B vitamins and also contain magnesium, selenium, and zinc, helpful.

Recent studies in Japan suggest that an extract of shiitaki mushrooms called sulfated B-glucans may have a beneficial effect against HIV. Much more research is needed, however, and currently there is no evidence that eating the mushrooms will help. Another mushroom extract, somastatin, may help improve the immune function of AIDS patients, but again, the research is very preliminary.

Researchers are also looking into hypericin, the active ingredient of the herb St. John's wort. This substance has an antiviral effect on mice and may be helpful for HIV and AIDS patients. However, St. John's wort tea has not been shown to help kill the virus.

Chronic diarrhea is a frequent problem for AIDS patients. Herbal treatments for diarrhea abound, but they are meant for the sort of minor, self-limiting diarrhea caused by occasional intestinal upsets. Diarrhea in AIDS patients is a serious matter that should not be self-treated. See your doctor.

❖ Alcoholism

Alcoholism is both a physical and psychological dependency on alcohol. Alcoholics drink in excess of the usual cultural limits and to the detriment of their physical health and social relationships. There are some ten million alcoholics in the United States, and many more people who drink heavily (more than two drinks a day).

Consumed heavily, alcohol damages many parts of the body, especially the liver. Virtually all alcoholics eventually suffer cirrhosis of the liver. In addition, alcoholism can cause chronic gastritis, pancreatitis, and weaken and damage the muscular tissue of the heart (cardiomyopathy). It can cause impotence in men; women who drink during pregnancy may cause birth defects in their babies. Alcohol is also a major cause of death and injuries due to accidents. About half of all traffic accidents involve alcohol.

Alcoholics often suffer from overall malnutrition, in part because alcohol depresses the appetite and in part because alcohol interferes with the body's ability to digest and absorb food. Alcoholics often suffer from serious deficiencies in vitamin C and vitamin B (particularly thiamine and B_{12}). Alcohol can also cause hypoglycemia, a sudden sharp drop in the blood sugar level that usually occurs a few hours after a period of heavy drinking. The drinker feels suddenly dizzy, weak, confused, and very hungry. Eating something sweet such as a jelly doughnut, cookies, or a candy bar can relieve the symptoms. These foods, like alcohol, have a lot of calories but little nutrition.

These health and nutrition problems can be treated as soon as the alcoholic stops drinking. Recovering alcoholics who have recently quit drinking are usually advised to eat a low-fat, high-calorie diet that is high in vitamins and minerals. Vitamin supplements can be very helpful during the recovery period. Alcoholics often have a deficiency of zinc, magnesium, and potassium. Experimental work with laboratory animals suggests that zinc deficiency due to excess alcohol consumption may trigger an increased desire for even more alcohol. Interestingly, although there is no evidence that a zinc deficiency in humans causes or affects alcoholism, many of the herbs traditionally recommended to recovering alcoholics to help restore liver function contain zinc and other vitamins and minerals often deficient in alcoholics. Dandelion, for example, has zinc, magnesium, niacin, and many B vitamins, including vitamin B_{12}. Kelp is another good source of all B vitamins. Goldenseal root and yellow dock have potassium; gotu kola has magnesium. Alfalfa, which is often recommended by naturopaths to detoxify the liver, is an excellent all-around source of vitamins, minerals, and other nutrients. Alfalfa can be taken in commercially prepared capsules or liquid or eaten as sprouts.

Silymarin, an antioxidant flavonoid found in milk thistle, may have a beneficial effect on the liver by stimulating the production of new liver cells. Because this could be especially helpful to patients suffering from cirrhosis, milk thistle is currently under active scientific investigation. Herbalists recommend that silymarin be taken in the form of milk thistle capsules, found in health food stores.

For treating the agitation, sleeplessness, and anxiety that often accompany withdrawal from alcohol, European doctors have long recommended valerian root. It seems to be most effective in the form of a tea or extract taken several times daily. Skullcap leaves, taken as a tea, are also helpful. Tea made from hops is reputed to help reduce the craving for alcohol.

❖ Allergies

An allergy is an abnormal sensitivity to a substance, such as pollen, that most people tolerate. An allergic reaction occurs when the body's natural defense system mistakenly identifies a substance (called an allergen) as harmful. In an attempt to protect the body, the defense system overreacts and produces chemicals in the blood that then produce allergic symptoms such as runny nose, wheezing, sneezing, itching, hives, or rashes. You have an allergy to a food or substance *only* if you have an immune system response. Any other sort of reaction is considered an intolerance, or even just a plain dislike.

Allergic reactions can vary considerably in their causes and effects. Respiratory allergies include hay fever (allergic rhinitis) and asthma. Common skin allergies include eczema (atopic dermatitis), hives (urticaria), and contact dermatitis. Food allergies, particularly to fish, eggs, milk, nuts, and wheat, are fairly common in young children and are often outgrown after age three.

In many cases, simply avoiding the known allergen, such as animal dander or shellfish, can reduce or eliminate allergic symptoms. Unfortunately, avoiding many allergens, such as mold or pollen, isn't always so easy. In many cases, you will simply have to treat the symptoms instead. Burdock, dandelion, garlic, onion, and goldenseal have been traditionally recommended as overall aids to reducing or relieving allergies. The effectiveness, if any, of these herbs varies considerably from person to person. One caveat: If you are allergic to pollen, avoid goldenseal, since it is a member of the ragweed family.

See also Asthma; Eczema; Hay Fever; Hives.

❖ Alzheimer's Disease

Alzheimer's disease (AD), a progressive, degenerative disease that attacks the brain and results in impaired memory, thinking, and behavior, is the most common cause of dementia in elderly people. Symptoms that signal the onset of Alzheimer's (usually after age sixty-five), include mild forgetfulness and confusion. As the disease progresses, confusion increases, and the patient becomes increasingly unable to carry out everyday tasks; later symptoms may include behavioral and personality changes, such as aggressive acts and aimless wandering. In the final stages of the disease, the Alzheimer's patient may require round-the-clock care.

The risk of Alzheimer's increases steadily with age. Some researchers estimate that as many as 3 percent of all people age sixty-five to seventy-four and half of all people over age eighty-five have the disease. These statistics add up to about four million people in the United States—including former president Ronald Reagan—currently suffering from Alzheimer's disease. Because the population is aging, an estimated fourteen million Americans will have AD by the year 2050. A recent study estimates that the cost of caring for one person with Alzheimer's disease is $47,000 a year, and most people with AD live for eight to twenty years after diagnosis.

Alzheimer's disease is named after Dr. Alois Alzheimer, the German psychiatrist who first described the condition in 1906. Dr. Alzheimer examined the brain tissue of a woman who had died of an unusual mental illness. He found abnormal deposits (plaques) and tangled bundles of nerve fibers. Plaques and tangles are now recognized as the characteristic abnormalities of the disease. In addition, victims of Alzheimer's disease have reduced amounts of the neurotransmitter chemicals vital for relaying complex messages among the nerve cells of the brain. Alzheimer's can be difficult to diagnose because other, treatable conditions, such as a brain tumor, can cause similar symptoms. Unfortunately, there is as yet no single diagnostic test for Alzheimer's disease.

Because concentrations of aluminum have been found in the brain plaques of some deceased AD patients, some researchers warned against the use of aluminum cookware and aluminum-containing deodorants. Later research, however, has shown that there's no evidence that aluminum, the third most common element on earth, causes Alzheimer's disease.

Other research has proven more encouraging. People with AD have low levels of the neurotransmitter called acetylcholine, which contains a substance related to vitamin B called choline. Since lecithin is a dietary source of choline, supplementing the diet of Alzheimer's patients with lecithin may be helpful in the early stages of the disease. So far, however, firm evidence is lacking. Many advanced Alzheimer's patients are deficient in vitamin B_{12} and other nutrients, but whether this is a cause or effect remains unknown. The fact is that there is little evidence to link Alzheimer's disease with dietary factors.

Some Alzheimer's patients are said to improve after consuming the herbs butcher's broom and ginkgo biloba (sometimes called maidenhair tree). Butcher's broom tops and seeds have traditionally been used to improve the circulation, which may help AD patients by increasing blood flow to their brains. Prepare it as a tea and give the patient 1 cup daily. Ginkgo biloba leaves also have a powerful effect on the circulatory system, particularly improving the blood flow to the brain. For Alzheimer's patients, herbalists usually recommend ginkgo biloba leaves in fluid extract form.

Herbs that are said to act as a general aid to mental alertness and longevity include ginseng, gotu kola, and sage. Traditional Chinese herbal medicine recommends 1/2 cup of ginseng tea three times daily. Herbalists suggest a tincture of gotu kola, recommending 15 to 30 drops three times a day. Sage is also said to help improve memory in the elderly.

Coping with a loved one who suffers from Alzheimer's disease is an exhausting, emotionally draining task that can impose severe physical and financial burdens on you. You are not alone—help of many kinds is available from:

Alzheimer's Association
919 North Michigan Avenue
Chicago, IL 60611-1676
800/272-3900

❖ Anemia

Anemia is a condition that occurs when your red blood cells don't contain enough hemoglobin, a protein that carries oxygen to your cells. Your cells are starved of oxygen, and as a result, you feel tired all the time, are short of breath, and may have a fast heartbeat. You might also be pale and irritable.

The most common cause of anemia is a shortage of iron in your blood, because you need iron to make hemoglobin. Iron-deficiency anemia can be caused by a lack of iron in the diet (especially if you diet a lot), by pregnancy, or by blood loss. Women who have very heavy menstrual periods can become anemic. Internal bleeding from an ulcer, ulcerative colitis, cancer, or other problems could also cause anemia. If blood loss is the cause of your anemia, it is extremely important for your doctor to find out why and treat the underlying problem.

Iron-deficiency anemia can usually be prevented and treated with a diet that is rich in iron and other nutrients. Foods high in iron include liver, seafood, nuts, beans, black-strap molasses, and dark green leafy vegetables such as spinach and kale. However, only about 10 percent of the iron in foods is actually absorbed by the body, so serious cases of iron-deficiency anemia may need treatment with supplemental iron pills. It's also important to get enough vitamin C in your diet. This will help your body absorb iron better from food.

Some herbs can be helpful for anemia. Yellow dock leaves and roots are rich in iron. In fact, an early American home remedy for anemia—a syrup of blackstrap molasses and yellow dock extract—can still be helpful today. Take 2 tablespoons daily. Dandelion leaves contain both iron and vitamin C. Stinging nettle is rich in iron and other valuable nutrients. Alfalfa is an excellent source of all vitamins and minerals. Avoid burdock root, however, since it can interfere with iron absorption.

Inadequate vitamin B_{12} or folic acid in the diet causes megaloblastic anemia. In this form of anemia, the red blood cells are large, fragile, and low in number. The effect is the same, however: your body is starved of oxygen. Vitamin B_{12} is found in animal foods such as lean meats, poultry, fish, milk, cheese, and eggs. Strict vegetarians who eat no dairy products or eggs can get their vitamin B_{12} from fermented soybean foods such as miso. Folic acid, which works in concert with vitamin B_{12} in the body, is found in many dietary sources, including leafy dark green vegetables (kale, spinach, romaine lettuce, and the like), liver, orange juice, avocados, beets, and broccoli. Brewer's yeast is another good source. Dong quai, a traditional Chinese herbal remedy, contains vitamin B_{12} as well as folic acid and is often recommended by herbalists to treat megaloblastic anemia. Alfalfa contains all the B vitamins and is said to be very helpful for this sort of anemia; dandelion leaves also contain many B vitamins, including vitamin B_{12}. Chickweed contains iron, vitamin C, and vitamin B_{12}.

Pernicious anemia is relatively rare and occurs when your body, for unknown reasons, stops absorbing vitamin B_{12} or folic acid. Pernicious anemia should not be self-treated. Your physician will recommend regular injections of vitamin B_{12} instead.

❖ Angina

Angina pectoris is dull, constricting pain in the center of the chest that occurs when the heart is temporarily starved of oxygen. Ordinarily, the arteries that supply oxygen-rich blood to your heart can easily handle any increased demand for blood flow due to exercise, cold temperatures, emotions, and so on. If the arteries are constricted or partially blocked, however, the heart muscle doesn't get the oxygen it needs. The result is angina. The pain usually goes away as the demand for oxygen lessens.

Because angina is usually a sign of coronary artery heart disease, it should be taken seriously. See your doctor as soon as possible if you experience anginalike symptoms, even if they last for only a few minutes. If you have angina and the symptoms are getting worse the situation could be urgent. See your doctor at once. You could be at serious risk of having a heart attack.

Diet and lifestyle changes can have a beneficial effect on angina. If you smoke, stop. Cut back on alcohol or eliminate it altogether. If you are overweight, discuss a weight loss plan with your doctor. In general, most physicians recommend a low-salt, low-fat, high-fiber diet and moderate exercise for angina patients, along with appropriate medication.

Some researchers believe that angina is linked to low levels of the fatty acid omega-3. Omega-3, or fish oil, is found in deep sea fish such as tuna, herring, and mackerel; it can also be purchased commercially in capsules. This point has become more controversial recently, however, when the results of a careful, long-term study indicated that eating fish more often did not prevent heart disease in men. Garlic and onions contain substances that help thin the blood. Since this can be helpful for angina patients, many doctors suggest they add garlic and onions to their daily diet in addition to taking their medication.

In Europe, an herbal remedy for angina based on hawthorn flowers and berries is commercially available. This remedy is not currently available in the United States, and it is unclear if hawthorn has a genuinely beneficial effect. Do not attempt to self-treat angina with hawthorn.

In traditional herbal medicine, various herbs are sometimes recommended as heart tonics. These include lobelia, lily of the valley, motherwort, and ginseng. Angina is a serious condition, however, and one that responds very well to lifestyle changes and standard drug therapy. Herbal medicine should not be used in place of proven treatments.

❖ Anorexia Nervosa

Anorexia nervosa, a refusal to eat that leads to severe weight loss, is a problem common among teenage American girls. Anorexics have a distorted view of the world and of themselves. They continue to feel that their bodies are too fat, even after they have lost more than 25 percent of their body weight. Anorexics become obsessed with compulsive exercising and losing weight, often starving themselves down to only 70 or 80 pounds.

The roots of anorexia are almost always psychological, and dietary measures alone probably won't help. Some researchers feel, however, that zinc deficiency may be among the underlying causes of the problem. Anorexics should be encouraged to eat or drink nourishing foods, preferably those that contain zinc, such as fish, milk, beef, whole grains, eggs, carrots, rice, and many others. Brewer's yeast is a good source of zinc; herbal sources include burdock root, dandelion leaves, garlic, horsetail stems, kelp, rose hips, and watercress leaves.

❖ Anxiety

Tension or apprehensiveness in the face of major stress is a perfectly normal form of anxiety. Sometimes anxiety can get out of control, however, leaving you feeling vaguely worried or fearful for no obvious reason. Sometimes the anxiety escalates into an overwhelming sense of dread and fear. Real physical symptoms accompany anxiety: tense muscles, shortness of breath, rapid heartbeat, dry mouth, inability to concentrate, and insomnia are the usual signs.

Some changes in your lifestyle and diet can help you get anxiety back under control. Relaxation techniques such as yoga, biofeedback, and deep breathing can help you control the symptoms. Regular exercise also helps reduce anxiety by inducing a feeling of well-being. Reduce or eliminate alcohol from your diet, and eliminate any substance abuse. Self-medicating with alcohol and drugs may be temporarily helpful, but in the long run they make you even more anxious and depressed.

Eliminating caffeine from your diet is probably the easiest and most important step you can take to help reduce anxiety. Caffeine is a powerful stimulant that is found not only in coffee and tea but in many soft drinks (even the ones that aren't cola flavored), and chocolate. Many over-the-counter medications such as diet pills and cold and cough medicines contain caffeine; read the labels.

A variety of herbs have been traditionally recommended for soothing anxiety. Valerian root, as an infusion or tincture, is a centuries-old sedative that remains very popular today. Passion flower is another traditional remedy, usually taken as a tea. Hops tea is another timeworn remedy for anxiety; it contains some of the same constituents as valerian and has a similar, though considerably less powerful, effect. Skullcap is traditionally recommended as a general relaxant and restorative. The leaves can be taken as a tea or tincture; the root is commercially available as a powder in capsules. Soothing teas of borage, lavender, and lemon balm are also recommended by herbalists. Teas of linden leaves, vervain, or wood betony may also be helpful for relieving anxiety, but avoid these herbs if you are pregnant. A flavorful combination for relieving anxiety is a mixture of skullcap, wood betony, lavender, and lemon balm. Mix the herbs together in whatever proportions you wish, and prepare them as an infusion; drink it hot.

Gamma-aminobutyric acid (GABA), an amino acid your body needs in small amounts, is sometimes recommended by herbalists and naturopaths as a treatment for anxiety; they usually suggest taking 750 milligrams of GABA daily. However, large doses of single amino acids are unlikely to have any desired effect and are potentially toxic. The Food and Drug Administration does not consider single amino acid supplements to be generally recognized as safe.

❖ Appetite Loss

In the case of a minor illness or injury to a normally healthy person, a few days of eating lightly or even not at all (as long as you take in plenty of fluids) won't do much harm. But in the case of chronic illness or serious injury, appetite loss can be a serious problem. Without good nutrition, the healing process is slowed, and the patient may become more susceptible to secondary infections. Appetite loss can also be a problem for depressed people and the elderly, who may lose interest in food or have difficulty eating. This could then lead to malnutrition, illness, and worsening of chronic conditions.

A traditional herbal approach to appetite loss is a variety of bitter herbs. These herbs can stimulate the flow of saliva in the mouth and gastric juices in the stomach, which is the body's way of saying, "I'm hungry." Gentian is one herb that is particularly effective as an appetite stimulant. (In fact, gentian is the principal flavoring in Angostura bitters, a mixture used in many apertifs, although the alcohol is probably the real appetite stimulant here.) To make gentian tea, boil 1 teaspoon of powdered gentian root in 1/2 cup of water for five minutes. Strain before drinking. Most herbalists recommend drinking the tea half an hour before mealtime; have no more than 2 cups daily. If gentian is not available, try substituting blessed thistle leaves. A cup of ginseng tea before meals is a traditional Chinese remedy for poor appetite.

Adding aromatic flavorings such as oregano, basil, garlic, cayenne pepper, rosemary, lemon juice, black pepper, and other favorite herbs and spices to bland food can make it tastier and more interesting. This is particularly helpful for the elderly and others whose appetite loss may be due to a dulled sense of taste.

❖ Arthritis

Over 100 rheumatic diseases affect the joints and other connective tissues of the body. By far the most common, however, are the two most usual forms of arthritis: osteoarthritis and rheumatoid arthritis.

Osteoarthritis

Osteoarthritis, also sometimes called degenerative arthritis, is the most common form of arthritis—nearly sixteen million Americans suffer from it. This type of arthritis occurs when the smooth layers of cartilage that act as a pad between the bones in a joint become thin, frayed, worn, or pitted. The result is pain, swelling, stiffness, and limited movement in the affected joints.

For some people, osteoarthritis is a hereditary disease. In most people, it is related to years of wear and tear on the joints, especially weight-bearing joints such as the hips and knees. That's why almost all older people develop some osteoarthritis, and many younger people and athletes do.

Osteoarthritis sufferers usually have periods of discomfort that are often followed by relatively symptomless periods. Over time, however, osteoarthritis tends to get progressively worse. There is no cure, but the disease can be managed by lifestyle and diet changes, along with medication, when appropriate. The first line of defense against arthritis is the nonsteroidal anti-inflammatory drugs (NSAIDs). These drugs, which include aspirin and ibuprofen, block the release of prostaglandins by the body. Since prostaglandins trigger inflammation, these drugs help reduce pain, swelling, and stiffness.

Perhaps because osteoarthritis is so common and so painful, an unusually large number of bogus treatments and "miracle cures" are available to desperate sufferers. Many people who try the treatments claim they get relief, but it must be remembered that their symptoms often get better and worse by themselves. For example, someone who drinks a cup of cider vinegar mixed with honey four times a day (a popular folklore treatment) might experience a temporary remission of symptoms that has nothing to do with the treatment but is almost certainly coincidence or the result of simultaneous medical treatment. (See page 34 for tips on how to spot quack remedies.) There is, however, some very preliminary evidence that omega-3 fatty acids (fish oil) can help relieve the symptoms of osteoarthritis. It is possible that the omega-3 fatty acids, like NSAIDs, block the body's production of prostaglandins. Discuss the use of omega-3 with your doctor before trying it.

Thus far, aside from the possible benefits of omega-3, *no* dietary regimen or nutritional supplement has been shown to relieve or prevent the symptoms of osteoarthritis, despite many clinical trials.

Traditional herbal remedies for osteoarthritis, a disease as old as humanity itself, have been used for centuries. One of the best-known and oldest herbal treatments is a tea made from powdered willow bark, which contains compounds closely related to salicylic acid, the principal component in aspirin. However, to obtain the equivalent relief of two standard aspirin tablets (325 milligrams each), you would have to drink well over a gallon of bitter-tasting tea, assuming a 7 percent concentration of active ingredients; and the willow bark sold in health food stores generally has just 1 percent. Even the capsule form would require you to take very large quantities, and you would have to wait several hours to feel the effect.

Like willow bark, meadowsweet is another herb that contains salicylates. It, too, has been recommended as a treatment for arthritic pain for centuries. Again, you would have to drink very large amounts of tea made from meadowsweet leaves to experience the relief two aspirin tablets bring. Meadowsweet is available as a tincture, but even in concentrated form, the dose would be more than any herbalist or physician would recommend. Dozens of other herbs, including alfalfa, black cohosh, blue-green algae, bog bean, burdock root, celery seeds, chapparal, comfrey, dandelion, devil's claw, feverfew, parsley, sassafras, valerian, and yucca, have been reputed to bring relief of arthritis. There is little or no evidence that any of them are effective.

External herbal treatments—an essential oil or cream that is rubbed into the skin at the affected joint or a hot herbal poultice or compress—are also often recommended and may provide some temporary relief. In general, these treatments do no harm, although some oils could cause skin irritation. Herbalists typically recommend wintergreen (menthol) oil, linseed oil, juniper oil, or borage oil as rubs for the aching joint; comfrey cream is often suggested. Hot compresses of angelica root tincture (also sometimes called by its Chinese name, dong quai), meadowsweet tincture, or diluted chickweed tincture are used to help relieve joint pain. However, the heat of the hot compress, not the herb tincture, is probably what provides the relief.

Some European physicians apply stinging nettle leaves to the skin at the site of the arthritic joint, supposedly relieving the joint pain through the application of a counterirritant. This treatment is very far from being proved effective, however, and the painful skin rash caused by the nettles could be as bad or worse than the arthritis. Similarly, there is no evidence whatsoever that bee stings on the skin at the painful joint will alleviate arthritis. All these treatments do is prove what lengths people will go to in their search for relief.

Self-Help for Osteoarthritis
Although your natural tendency is to stay off painful joints, physicians agree that it is important for people with osteoarthritis to stay as active as possible. Inactivity can lead to weakened and stiff muscles, further restricting your range of motion; in turn, weak muscles make it even harder to get around, causing more pain in the joints and deepening the discomfort cycle. Try exercising in small amounts throughout the day, with rest periods in between. Exercises that don't strain the joints are best. Water exercise, also called aquacise, is easiest on your joints, because much of your body's weight is supported by the water. Water exercise programs designed for arthritic people are often offered at com-

munity centers with swimming pools, such as your local YMCA or high school.

One good way to reduce osteoarthritis symptoms is to lose weight if you are too heavy. If you are overweight, your joints have to carry the extra pounds, adding to the strain on them. This can make your arthritis get worse faster.

Rheumatoid Arthritis

Rheumatoid arthritis is a chronic inflammatory disease that causes pain, stiffness, swelling, deformity, and permanent loss of function in the affected joints. In addition, sufferers may have general symptoms such as fatigue, weakness, and loss of appetite. Rheumatoid arthritis is one of the most severe forms of arthritis. It affects over two million Americans, two-thirds of whom are women.

As discussed above, a few preliminary studies suggest that omega-3 fatty acids (found in fish oil) may relieve some rheumatoid arthritis symptoms. Other small, preliminary studies suggest that gamma-linolenic acid (GLA), a component of unsaturated fats found in plants such as black currant, borage, and evening primrose, could reduce joint inflammation. However, the amounts needed are very high, far more than ordinary supplements could supply. There is also some evidence, although it is largely anecdotal, that eating fresh ginger can relieve rheumatoid arthritis symptoms. If you are being treated for rheumatoid arthritis, discuss these remedies with your doctor before trying them. Recent studies show that certain antibiotics might be effective in relieving the symptoms of rheumatoid arthritis.

Some victims of rheumatoid arthritis claim that specific foods such as milk and dairy products cause or worsen their symptoms. Others claim that foods from the nightshade family, including tomatoes, potatoes, eggplant, and bell peppers, make their arthritis worse. Still others believe that meat, especially cured meats such as bacon, bring on flareups of symptoms. Carefully controlled studies have shown, however, that a clear cause and effect relationship between eating a specific food and having symptoms is actually quite rare. There is very little evidence that eliminating certain foods, going on a vegetarian diet, or avoiding milk products or meat will have any effect on arthritis.

Arthritis Quackery

The Arthritis Foundation suggests these tips to help you spot questionable arthritis remedies.

A remedy is bogus if it:

- Cures all kinds of arthritis
- Uses case histories and testimonials
- Cites only one study
- Cites a study that has no control group
- Comes without directions for use
- Doesn't list contents on the label
- Has no warning about side effects
- Is described as harmless or natural
- Is based on a secret formula
- Claims it cures arthritis
- Is available only from one source
- Is promoted only in the media, in books, or by mail
- Is sold only be mail order

See also Gout; Lupus Erythematosus.

❖ Asthma

Periodic attacks of wheezing and difficulty breathing are the classic symptoms of asthma, a chronic inflammatory condition of the lungs. If you have asthma, the airways of your lungs are unusually sensitive to airborne allergens (such as pollen) and irritants (such tobacco, smoke, air pollution, or chalk dust). Some asthma sufferers are also sensitive to certain foods. When you are exposed to any of these substances—asthma triggers—the linings of the airways swell up; this narrows the airways and makes it hard for you to breathe. The muscles that surround the airways can then go into spasms, which makes breathing even harder. The inflamed linings of your airways also produce mucus, which clogs them up. These reactions combine to make breathing very difficult. In addition, you might feel a painless tightening in your chest and wheeze, sometimes very noticeably, when you breathe.

About 5 percent of asthmatics are sensitive to the salicylates found in certain foods and some medications such as aspirin and other nonsteroidal anti-inflammatory drugs, and to sulfites, which are widely used as preservatives in foods and beverages. Foods that naturally contain salicylates include tea, root beer, corned beef, avocados, cucumbers, green peppers, olives, potatoes, tomatoes, apples, berries, cherries, grapes, melons, peaches, and plums. The herbs willow bark, meadowsweet, cowslip/primrose (or primula), chamomile, lady's mantle, yarrow, red clover flowers, and sweet violet/heartsease (or viola) also contain salicylates and should be avoided. Since other, less common herbs may contain salicylates, people with this sensitivity should simply avoid all herbal remedies to be on the safe side. Sulfites are commonly used in restaurants and convenience foods to help preserve the freshness of shrimp, potatoes, dehydrated soups, and many other foods. They are also found naturally in beer, wine, and dried fruits (especially apricots). Monosodium glutamate (MSG), another widely used food preservative, can also trigger asthma attacks in sensitive individuals. Asthmatics who are sensitive to sulfites or MSG should be very careful to avoid these ingredients.

Some asthma attacks are triggered by a food. The most common culprits are milk, eggs, seafood, chocolate, and nuts.

Most asthmatics require drug treatment under medical supervision to control their attacks. In addition to their drug treatment, however, asthmatics may be able to help themselves have fewer and less severe attacks by adding some foods to their diets.

Because the underlying cause of an asthma attack is inflammation of the airways, eating onions, which have nat-

ural anti-inflammatory properties, may help. It's possible
that quercetin and thiosulfinate, two compounds found in
onions, are responsible. Eating a lot of hot, spicy foods, such
as chili peppers and strong mustard, can help thin the mucus
that clogs airways.

The caffeine in coffee can also help asthmatics avoid attacks and relieve the symptoms. In general, people who regularly drink 3 cups of coffee a day are markedly less likely
to have asthma. If you're having an attack, 2 cups of strong
coffee can help relieve your symptoms. This is probably because the caffeine in the coffee contains a substance called
theophylline, which helps relax muscle spasms around the
airways. In fact, theophylline by itself is a commonly prescribed asthma drug. It's not a good idea to substitute coffee
for your regular asthma medication, however. Since asthma
can be deadly, self-help steps should never take the place of
medical supervision.

Many herbal remedies have been suggested for asthma
over the centuries, but only one has any proven beneficial effect: ephedra, also known by its Chinese name ma huang.
Ephedra has traditionally been used as an asthma medication
in China and India for thousands of years. Ephedra contains
ephedrine and other related alkaloids that relieve bronchial
spasm; the synthetic form is found in some prescription
asthma medications. Herbalists generally recommend drinking a tea made from 1 heaping teaspoon of ephedra steeped
in 16 ounces of boiling water for ten minutes. This dosage is
usually effective for relieving asthma symptoms. The draw-
backs are obvious, however: Time is needed to prepare the
mixture, you have to drink a lot of it, and it takes some time
to work. In addition, large doses can cause nervousness,
headaches, dizziness, and other side effects that are unpleasant in general and could be dangerous if you also have high
blood pressure, diabetes, a heart condition, or some other
chronic problem. If you have an asthma attack, treat it
promptly with the medicine your doctor advises.

Although the North American herb Mormon tea, also
sometimes called squaw tea, desert herb, or Brigham Young
weed, is a species of ephedra, it does not contain any of the

alkaloid substances found in ma huang and has no effect on asthma.

Other herbs that are traditionally recommended for asthma include thorn apple, thyme, yerba santa, coltsfoot, elecampane root, wild cherry bark, valerian, chickweed, fenugreek seeds, and lobelia. None have been shown to be effective, so don't try to treat asthma with them.

❖ Atherosclerosis

Atherosclerosis, the medical term for fatty plaque buildup on the walls of the arteries leading to the heart, occurs gradually and has no one single cause. This condition causes these crucial blood vessels to become narrowed or even blocked. The result is coronary artery disease: angina or a heart attack. Two major factors are closely associated with atherosclerosis: high levels of blood cholesterol and high levels of a blood-clotting protein called fibrinogen. By reducing the levels of these two factors through diet and medication where appropriate, you may be able to prevent or lessen atherosclerosis.

A healthy lifestyle can play an important role in treating atherosclerosis. Risk factors that can be controlled include cigarette smoking, obesity, high blood pressure, diabetes, and lack of exercise. Statistically, sex, age, race, and heredity are all uncontrollable factors that play a part: men have more heart attacks than women; the risk of heart attack increases with age; African-American men are most likely of all to have heart attacks; and atherosclerosis runs in families.

There are many dubious claims for herbs that supposedly dissolve arterial plaque. Although garlic has been shown to help reduce high cholesterol levels, which slows or possibly halts further plaque, it does not remove existing plaque. The same may be true of oolong tea. Ginkgo biloba, hawthorn berries, and chickweed, despite claims, do not remove cholesterol buildups from the arteries. Atherosclerosis is a serious condition. Don't attempt to treat it yourself.

See also Angina; Heart Attack; High Cholesterol.

❖ Athlete's Foot

Athlete's foot (tinea pedis) is caused by a fungal infection that lodges itself into the warm, moist area between your toes, especially the webbing between the fourth and fifth (little) toes. The itching, redness, scaling, burning, blistering, and oozing of athlete's foot is annoying, uncomfortable, and persistent.

Prevention is the best treatment for athlete's foot. Good hygiene and keeping your feet dry are the most important preventive measures. Wash your feet daily with soap and water. Dry them thoroughly with a clean towel, being sure to dry between the toes. Let your feet air for five to ten minutes before putting on socks, stockings, or shoes. Some people find that a light dusting of talcum powder on the feet helps absorb moisture; herbalists sometimes recommend powdered hemlock bark instead (this product is not usually carried in health food stores, however). If your feet sweat heavily, disposable, absorbent insoles placed in your shoes may help. Materials that do not breathe (nylon and other synthetic materials, for example) trap moisture on the feet, creating a breeding ground for fungus. Whenever possible, wear absorbent socks made of natural fiber and lightweight shoes that freely encourage air circulation. Change shoes frequently so that moisture doesn't build up in them.

Athlete's foot was a scourge of the ancient Romans, and their traditional herbal recipes to relieve the symptoms have been handed down for over two thousand years. There's no real evidence that any herbs kill the fungus, but ointments made from calendula or aloe vera can relieve the discomfort. Soaking your feet in a footbath containing a decoction made from goldenseal is another traditional remedy. Use 1 teaspoon of ground goldenseal root per cup of boiling water; let the mixture cool until it is just hot before you soak your feet. Alternatively, add 1 teaspoon of goldenseal tincture per cup of hot water.

Australian tea tree oil has an antifungal effect. Apply the oil sparingly to the affected area in the morning and again before going to sleep. Tea tree oil helps relieve the itching and could help you get rid of your athlete's foot completely if applied for several weeks.

If you have diabetes or circulatory problems, see your doctor if you develop the symptoms of athlete's foot. Also see your doctor if your foot symptoms include white, soggy tissue; oozing; very severe itching; or foot odor.

❖ Bad Breath

Most cases of bad breath (halitosis) are temporary and caused by what you eat or drink. Pungent foods such as onions, garlic, salami, canned fish, and strong cheeses leave odorous, sulfur-containing compounds behind in your mouth. Coffee and alcoholic beverages, especially wine, beer, and whiskey, also leave a long-lasting residue. This sort of bad breath lasts until the noxious compounds dissipate, which could take up to twenty-four hours, depending on how much you ate. Fortunately, bad breath can be sweetened the traditional way. Try chewing on a few fennel or anise seeds, some fresh parsley sprigs, fresh mint or thyme leaves, or some cloves.

Mouthwashes are effective, but only temporarily. Most commercial mouthwashes contain alcohol along with eucalyptol, menthol, or thymol as flavoring. You can make your own, nonalcoholic mouthwash by diluting 1 part eucalyptus oil, peppermint oil, thyme oil, or tea tree oil in 10 parts water. Myrrh is another natural remedy often recommended for oral hygiene. It tastes terrible, but it can be effective. Try making a mouthwash out of 1 part myrrh oil diluted in 15 parts water.

A more serious cause of bad breath is poor oral hygiene. Bacteria in your mouth give off the same sort of sulfurous compounds as garlic. Dentists recommend brushing your teeth after every meal to remove the bacteria that could cause bad breath. If you can't brush, try rinsing your mouth with fresh water a few times after meals. Floss your teeth daily to remove food particles stuck between your teeth. Bacteria from the particles may be the culprit. You could also try gently brushing your tongue to remove food particles and bacteria there.

Persistent bad breath can be a symptom of more serious health problems, such as diabetes, cirrhosis of the liver, kidney failure, chronic sinusitis, dehydration, or gastrointestinal trouble. Drugs such as penicillin and lithium can cause bad breath, too. In about a third of all cases, however, persistent bad breath is caused by gum disease, which needs professional treatment.

See also Gum Disease, Tooth Care.

❖ Benign Breast Disease

Benign breast disease, also sometimes called fibrocystic breast disease or cystic mastitis, is so common among women that it really shouldn't be called a disease at all. Many women have breasts that are naturally lumpy and have a tendency to swell and become tender before menstruation. The breasts of older women often become lumpy as a normal part of the aging process.

The discomfort of breast swelling and tenderness can be relieved with some simple self-help steps. A good support bra helps quite a bit, as do over-the-counter nonsteroidal anti-inflammatory drugs such as aspirin and ibuprofen. Avoid nonprescription and herbal diuretics. They do help reduce breast swelling, but they can throw off your body's overall fluid balance and cause more problems than they solve. Ice packs also help some women.

Reducing your salt intake can also help lessen breast swelling and tenderness. Many women say that eliminating caffeine from their diet relieves their symptoms, sometimes dramatically. This has been extensively studied and never proved, but is certainly worth trying. Remember that caffeine is found not only in coffee and tea but also in soft drinks (especially colas), chocolate, and many over-the-counter and prescription medications.

Adding a vitamin E supplement to your diet might help reduce breast lumpiness, according to recent studies. Try taking one 400 IU vitamin E capsule daily.

Many women with fibrocystic breast disease also have low levels of selenium. Increasing your selenium intake to 100 micrograms daily could help your symptoms. The best sources of selenium are organ meats, seafood, lean meat, poultry, and whole grains such as oatmeal and brown rice. Interestingly, kelp, which is traditionally recommended for tender breasts, is also high in selenium along with many other useful vitamins and minerals. Try taking it in tablet form (available at health food stores) once or twice a day. Kelp is high in iodine, so discuss using it with your doctor if you are being treated for a thyroid condition.

Some women find that taking evening primrose oil supplements helps relieve their breast soreness. This may work because the oil contains gamma-linolenic acid, which your body needs to make prostaglandins, hormonelike substances that mediate a number of physiological processes, including inflammation and swelling. Try taking two capsules a day (2 grams) for two weeks before your period.

In almost all cases, the lumps of benign breast disease are not indicators or precursors of breast cancer, and having benign breast disease does not necessarily mean that your risk of breast cancer is increased. The lumps can make self-examination for cancerous lumps more difficult, however. If you have lumpy breasts, be sure to see your doctor regularly and have mammograms as recommended.

See also Breast Cancer; Premenstrual Syndrome (PMS).

❖ Bladder Infections
See Urinary Tract Infections.

❖ Blood Clots

When a blood clot (thrombus) forms in an already narrowed artery, it can block the flow of blood through the vessel. If the artery leads to the heart, a heart attack (myocardial infarction) can occur. If the artery leads to the brain, a stroke may result. Your tendency to form blood clots depends on how likely your blood platelets are to clump together, how much blood fibrinogen (a protein your body uses to make clots) you have, and how active your body's natural clot-dissolving system is.

A number of well-documented studies show that what you eat can have a big effect on how your blood clots. Substances in some foods and herbs can reduce your chances of a blood clot by making your platelets less sticky, making your blood less viscous (thinner), changing your fibrinogen levels, and helping your body dissolve clots when they form.

Onions and garlic can help block platelet clumping and thin the blood. A substance called quercetin in onions may be responsible. Garlic contains a compound called ajoene, which seems to have clot-busting effects. Both onions and garlic also contain adenosine, which has a blood-thinning effect. Many cardiologists now recommend that their patients eat an onion and a few cloves of garlic (raw or cooked) every day.

Onions and garlic also help reduce clotting by blocking the body's production of a prostaglandin called thromboxane, which makes your platelets clump together. Some other foods that reduce thromboxane production are ginger, cloves, turmeric, and cumin. A special type of black mushroom found in Chinese cuisine, the tree ear, may also have anticlotting effects. Like onions and garlic, this fungus contains adenosine. Coumarins, blood-thinning substances found naturally in licorice, citrus fruits, and some other foods, may also help protect against blood clots.

The omega-3 fatty acids found in fish can have a potent effect on blood clot formation. Omega-3 reduces platelet stickiness, lowers fibrinogen levels, and improves clot dissolving. Good sources of omega-3 fatty acids are fatty ocean fish such as tuna, herring, salmon, mackeral, and sardines. One gram of omega-3 fatty acids daily may be enough to reduce the chances of a blood clot by almost half. A daily 3- to 6-ounce serving of fatty fish will easily supply two or more grams.

Another food that may protect against blood clots is olive oil. Studies indicate that a daily dose of about 2 tablespoons of olive oil can help keep the platelets from clumping.

What you drink can also affect how your blood clots. The chemicals found in black and green tea (especially the Chinese variety called oolong) may reduce your platelet stickiness, thin your blood, and improve your clot-dissolving abilities. Exactly how these work is still under study; researchers suspect that the tannin in the tea plays a role.

A glass or two of red wine every day may also reduce your chances of a blood clot. A moderate amount of red wine seems to reduce platelet stickiness while also increasing HDL ("good") cholesterol levels in the blood. Scientists think that a compound called resveratrol is responsible. Since resveratrol is found in grape skins, red wine has it, but white wine doesn't (the skins are discarded when white wine is made).

If you are already taking any blood-thinning medications or have a history of bleeding problems, be sure to consult your physician before adding any clot-busting foods or supplements to your diet. Don't use the herb feverfew if you take blood-thinning drugs.

❖ Boils

A boil forms when you get a bacterial infection of a hair follicle. At first, the follicle is inflamed, red, and tender. After a few days, the red lump formed by the infection grows larger, fills with white or yellow pus, and becomes even more tender. Within the next few days, the pus usually bursts through the skin, draining the boil. After this, the boil gradually heals and disappears, generally within a week or two.

Since a boil is most painful before it drains, using hot compresses to help bring the boil to a head can reduce the period of discomfort quite a bit. To make a compress, place a clean washcloth or gauze pad soaked in hot water against the boil for fifteen or twenty minutes at a time, several times a day. Continue the treatment for a few days after the boil drains to keep it draining. Before the boil opens, try applying chickweed ointment between compress applications. Once the boil bursts, many herbalists recommend using a strong tea made from goldenseal root and echinacea root instead of a plain hot water compress; the astringency of the goldenseal helps keep the boil open and draining, while the echinacea root has natural antibiotic properties.

Boils are usually caused by infection from a *staphylococcus* bacteria, so it is important to keep the area around the boil clean with soap and water to avoid reinfecting yourself or passing the infection on to others. Wash your hands thoroughly before handling food, for example. You could also try taking echinacea internally while you have the boil.

Herbalists generally recommend two 200-milligram capsules a day to fight infections.

Recurrent boils can be a symptom of a more serious problem such as diabetes, so see your doctor if you get them often.

❖ Breast Cancer

Breast cancer statistics are pretty grim. Every year some 180,000 women are diagnosed with the disease and about 45,000 die from it. Over her entire lifetime, a woman has about a one in nine chance of getting breast cancer. The good news is that while breast cancer remains the most common type of cancer affecting American women, the death rate has dropped perceptibly over the past several years (by almost 5 percent from 1989 to 1992) and is likely to keep dropping as early detection and treatment methods continue to improve.

Risk Factors for Breast Cancer

There are several well-documented factors that increase the risk of breast cancer:

Age. Breast cancer is uncommon in women under the age of thirty-five. The risk increases as a woman grows older. Most breast cancers occur in women over the age of fifty; the risk is especially high for women over age sixty.

Family history. The risk of getting breast cancer increases for a woman whose mother, sister, or daughter has had the disease.

Personal history. About 15 percent of women treated for breast cancer get a second breast cancer later on.

Hormonal history. Factors related to your body's normal production of hormones can increase your breast cancer risk. These include early menstruation (before age twelve); late menopause (after age fifty-five); late first child (after age thirty); childlessness.

Diet. Breast cancer may be more likely among women who eat a high-fat diet or who are overweight.

The above high-risk factors are found in only about 25 percent of the women who develop breast cancer. In most cases, however, no particular risk factors—aside from being a woman and growing older—can be identified. Early detection through breast self-examination, regular checkups, and mammography remain the most reliable ways to find breast cancer at its beginning stages, when treatment is most likely to be effective.

Dietary Fat and Breast Cancer

The merits of a low-fat diet for helping to prevent breast cancer have been extensively studied. Some convincing studies have shown that there is a high association between dietary fat and breast cancer, but as yet no direct link has been shown. A recent study of Greek women, however, suggests that a diet high in fresh fruits and vegetables and olive oil has a protective effect against the disease. Paradoxically, the women in the study had a high intake of total fat (higher than what doctors recommend), but probably because most of it came from monounsaturated olive oil, the risk of breast cancer was 25 percent lower among the postmenopausal women.

The Role of Estrogen

Some forms of breast cancer grow faster in the presence of the female hormones estrogen and progesterone. It's possible that high levels of these hormones may trigger breast cancer later in life. Obese women are somewhat more likely to get breast cancer, perhaps because being overweight stimulates the production of estrogen. Losing weight, then, is one possible way to decrease your estrogen levels. Another way may be to increase your consumption of cruciferous vegetables such as cabbage and broccoli; indoles (antioxidant compounds) in these foods could help speed up your body's metabolization of estrogen. Other possible estrogen-blocking compounds are found in wheat bran, beans, and soybean products such as tofu, soy milk, and miso. Alfalfa sprouts may also block estrogen.

The drug tamoxifen, which is derived from substances found in the bark of the Pacific yew tree, has been used to treat some cases of estrogen-dependent breast cancer, although its primary use is treating ovarian cancer. Tamoxifen is not an herbal treatment. Most parts of trees in the yew family are poisonous. Drinking or consuming any sort of herbal product based on yew will not help breast cancer (or anything else) and could be dangerous. Teas, tinctures, or ointments of red clover flowers are occasionally recommended by herbalists as a treatment for breast cancer. This is a worthless remedy that no responsible health care provider should ever suggest. If you think you might have breast cancer, see your doctor at once. Modern treatments have an excellent chance of success.

See also Benign Breast Disease; Chemotherapy; Radiation Therapy.

❖ Breast-Feeding

A mother can give her baby good, natural nutrition from the very start by breast-feeding. Nursing mothers need to eat at least 500 more calories a day than usual and need to drink lots of fluids. In general, a well-balanced diet that includes plenty of fruits and vegetables, whole grain cereals and bread, meat, beans, and milk and other dairy foods such as yogurt and cheese will supply the nutrition you need. Water or fruit juice such as orange juice, prune juice, and cider are all good choices. Good nutrition keeps you healthy and ensures a good flow of milk for your baby.

Nursing mothers also need extra calcium—1,200 milligrams a day—as well as extra vitamins and minerals, especially vitamin C, folic acid, and iron. Your doctor will probably recommend a daily multivitamin and calcium and iron supplements.

Caffeine, alcohol, amphetamines, barbiturates, and recreational drugs must be avoided, since these substances can get into your milk and be passed on to your baby. For the same reason, it's also important to avoid most medications, even nonprescription products such as acetaminophen (Tylenol), antihistamines, aspirin, cough syrups, and decongestants. Herbal medications generally contain much lower concentrations of active ingredients than prescription or nonprescription drugs, but even these should be avoided. Nursing mothers who use birth control pills should talk to their doctors about switching to a low-dosage pill containing only progestin.

Nursing mothers often worry about having an adequate flow of milk. The best way to increase your milk supply is to eat right, drink lots of fluids, get plenty of rest, not smoke, and nurse your baby often—nursing stimulates you to produce more milk. Traditionally, herbal teas made from fennel, anise, caraway, cumin, dill, or fenugreek seeds have been recommended to women to increase their milk supply. These teas are flavorful and mild, but drinking more of any liquid will probably have the same positive effect. A tea made from equal parts blessed thistle tops, red raspberry leaves, and marshmallow roots is another old-fashioned herbal remedy, but again, the positive effect is probably due to drinking more liquid. Borage leaf tea or comfrey tea are sometimes recommended by herbalists, but these should be avoided because of the high levels of toxic alkaloids they may contain.

Sore or cracked nipples are another problem for nursing mothers. Some women find that rubbing vitamin E oil into their nipples is soothing. An herbal ointment made with calendula in a lanolin or petroleum jelly base may be worth trying. Avoid herbal ointments made with comfrey. Anything used on your nipples should be washed off before feeding your baby.

❖ Bronchitis

Bronchitis is an inflammation of the mucus membranes lining the airways (bronchi) leading to your lungs. Symptoms of bronchitis include a deep cough that brings up yellowish or grayish phlegm from your lungs, wheezing, fever, and breathlessness.

Acute bronchitis is usually the result of a viral respiratory infection such as a bad cold or the flu. Generally, this clears up within a few days. If it doesn't, call your doctor.

A productive cough (one that brings up mucus) is the main sympton of bronchitis. Therefore, anything that thins the mucus and makes it easier to cough up will help. Moist, warm air is effective. Try using a vaporizer, breathing warm steam from a shower, or putting your head under a towel with a bowl of hot water. Eucalyptus oil or peppermint oil added to the water in the vaporizer gives off a pleasant aroma that could also help soothe your inflamed bronchial passages.

If you have a productive cough from bronchitis, be sure to drink *lots* of fluids—six to eight glasses a day of plain water, herbal teas, or fruit juice will help thin the mucus. Herbal teas with expectorant qualities can help you cough up the mucus in your airways. Two herbs in particular are often recommended for bronchitis: horehound and thyme. Horehound is a traditional early American remedy still popular today, in part because it has a pleasant flavor. Although the Food and Drug Administration no longer allows manufacturers to use horehound in nonprescription cough medicines, it does consider the herb to be generally recognized as safe, and allows nonprescription horehound cough lozenges to be sold. You can make horehound tea yourself using 2 heaping teaspoonfuls of dried leaves in 8 ounces of boiling water. Let it steep for five minutes and drink no more than 5 cups a day.

Thyme contains an oil that helps loosen mucus in your airways and helps relieve bronchospasm. To make thyme tea, place 1 to 2 heaping teaspoonfuls of dried leaves in 8 ounces of boiling water. Let steep for five minutes and drink no more than 3 cups a day.

Chronic bronchitis—bronchitis symptoms that persist or get worse—can be a serious medical condition that can lead to emphysema, pneumonia, heart failure, and other life-threatening medical problems. Although air pollution can be a cause of chronic bronchitis, the chief cause is cigarette smoking. If you smoke, stop. If you have chronic bronchitis, discuss any herbal remedies with your doctor before you try them.

❖ Bruising

Painful bruises occur when an internal blood vessel is damaged, allowing blood to seep into the surrounding tissues. The bruised area may be slightly swollen and tender to the touch, and will turn a dark black or blue color at first. Over a week or ten days, the color will gradually change and lighten as the bruise fades away.

A good way to relieve the discomfort and swelling of a bruise is to apply a cold compress or ice pack to the area, preferably soon after the injury. Leave the ice pack in place for ten to fifteen minutes; this is especially effective for bruises on the shin, scalp, or around the eye, which can swell up alarmingly at first.

A traditional herbal favorite for relieving bruise discomfort is arnica, in ointment or tincture form. If you use the tincture form, dilute it in 5 parts cold water first. Apply the arnica directly to the bruised area. Don't use arnica on broken skin, however, and if skin irritation develops, stop using it. Calendula ointment is another often-recommended remedy.

If you bruise more easily or frequently than normal, or if your bruises seem to last a long time, see your doctor. It might be an indication of a more serious problem such as a low level of blood platelets, leukemia, hemophilia, or AIDS.

But don't be alarmed. The problem is far more likely to be caused by a medication you are taking. Aspirin, blood thinners, asthma medicines, and steroids, among other medications, can cause you to bruise easily. If you think a prescription or nonprescription medication is causing your bruising, discuss it with your doctor.

Another possible cause of excess bruising could be too many omega-3 fatty acid (fish oil) supplements. The most likely dietary cause of bruising is a lack of vitamin C. Your body needs vitamin C to build strong blood vessels, and a shortage can lead to blood vessels that are easily damaged. Many doctors suggest adding 1,000 to 1,500 milligrams of vitamin C to the diet daily to combat bruising.

Another possible cause of bruising is a deficiency of vitamin K, which is essential for proper clotting. This sort of deficiency is quite rare, however, and is usually found only in people with serious intestinal diseases. Alfalfa, corn silk, gotu kola, and slippery elm bark are herbs that contain vitamin K, but the amounts are not sufficient to treat a serious dificiency. Treatment with supplemental vitamin K should be done only under medical supervision.

❖ Burns

Eighty percent of burn injuries occur in the home and many are related to cooking. Most of these accidents could be prevented by common sense and simple safety precautions: using pot holders, keeping matches and lighters away from children, not smoking in bed (preferably not smoking at all), not leaving hot irons unattended, and so on.

Doctors classify burns by their degree of severity. First-degree burns are minor burns that affect only the surface of the skin. These burns are red and painful, but the skin is not blistered (most sunburns are first-degree burns). These burns generally heal in three to four days and leave no scar. Second-degree burns are more serious because they affect the skin surface and the tissue just below it. These burns are characterized by redness, blisters, oozing, and more severe pain. Minor second-degree burns generally heal in about three weeks and leave no scar. Severe second-degree burns can take a month or more to heal and can leave thick scars. Third- and fourth-degree burns are severe burns that affect the tissue layers beneath the skin surface and the tissue beneath that.

In general, you can treat first-degree burns and minor second-degree burns yourself, with the following exceptions: if the burn covers an area larger than 1 percent of your body (approximately the size of the back of your hand); if it is a deep burn; any burn on the face or genital region; and burns affecting infants, children, the elderly, diabetics, or someone with a chronic illness. If any of the exceptions apply, see your doctor at once.

For minor burns, prompt treatment with cold-water therapy reduces or even eliminates the pain, redness, and swelling. Immediately run cold (not icy) water over the burned area. Continue until the pain stops—as long as 45 minutes, if necessary. Don't use an ice pack. Often, cold-water therapy is so effective that no other treatment is necessary. If serious burns are involved, begin cold-water therapy and call for medical help at once.

Old folk remedies such as putting honey, butter, or bacon grease on a burn are worse than useless. They will keep the heat in and make the burn worse, as well as providing a fertile ground for later infection. Once a minor burn is treated promptly with cold water, you don't really have to do anything else except to keep the area clean and dry. After a few days, soothe any lingering discomfort with fresh aloe vera gel or vitamin E oil. Applying lavender oil, calendula ointment, or arnica ointment may also help. If blisters develop, cover the area with clean gauze, but don't break the blisters, and don't use any sort of ointment on them. Do watch them, though. If pus, oozing, or red streaks develop, you have an infection and should see a doctor at once.

❖ Bursitis

Sacs filled with a lubricating fluid protect and cushion the cartilage and bones in joints such as your shoulder, knee, elbow, and hip. If these sacs, called bursas, become inflamed and swell up, you get the painful condition known as bursitis.

Bursitis is usually caused by an injury to the joint, often from sports or a repetitive motion, such as frequently kneeling down and getting up again (housemaid's knee). Generally, the best treatment is to rest the area and take a nonsteroidal anti-inflammatory drug such as aspirin or ibuprofen to reduce the swelling. Because bursitis has many of the same symptoms as arthritis, many herbalists advise the same traditional treatments. Most of these treatments, such as drinking willow bark tea or cherry juice or applying a cider vinegar compress, are not effective. Rubbing the skin at the affected joint with eucalyptus oil, menthol, or ginger juice may provide some temporary relief because of the counterirritation. If skin irritation develops, however, stop the treatment.

Some people find that an ice pack helps if the area is hot and swollen. After the swelling has gone down, heat from a heating pad sometimes brings relief. The pain and swelling often clear up by themselves in a week or two. If they don't, or if the pain and swelling are severe, see your doctor.

See also Arthritis.

❖ Cancer

Cancer occurs when cells in your body become abnormal and start to divide and form more cells without control or order. As the abnormal cells grow, they destroy body tissue. One out of every three Americans will get some form of cancer in their lifetime, and one out of every five cases will be fatal.

Cancer is a general term for a group of more than one hundred different diseases. Skin cancer is the most common type of cancer for both men and women. The next most common type among men is prostate cancer; among women, it is breast cancer. Lung cancer, however, is the leading cause of death from cancer for both men and women in the United States. Even though the incidence of cancer is rising, there's plenty of evidence to show that a change in your diet and lifestyle now can help reduce your chances of getting cancer later.

In many cases, no one really knows why someone gets a particular type of cancer. Specific risk factors such as age, heredity, smoking, obesity, and alcohol consumption increase your chances of getting some types, however. For example, 85 percent of all lung cancer patients smoke cigarettes, and smokers are twice as likely to get bladder cancer. Heavy drinking sharply increases the risk of cancer of the mouth, throat, esophagus, and larynx; if you both drink and smoke, the odds are even greater. Serious obesity appears to be linked to increased rates of cancer of the esophagus, prostate, pancreas, uterus, colon, and ovary; it may also be linked to breast cancer in older women.

The Anticancer Diet

Researchers at the National Cancer Institute estimate that about 35 percent of all cancers are related to diet, while some other researchers place the figure as high as 70 percent. Eating a healthy diet offers no guarantees, however—you can only reduce the odds, not eliminate them. Furthermore, the National Cancer Institute points out that there is no evidence that any kind of diet or food can either cure cancer or stop it from coming back.

So what should you eat to prevent cancer? In general, doctors recommend a diet that is low in fat and high in fresh fruits and vegetables. Strong evidence points to links between a high-fat diet and certain cancers, including cancer of the breast, colon, uterus, and prostate. Numerous studies have shown that people who eat lots of fresh fruits and vegetables have lower cancer rates than those who don't. How much is a lot? Two servings a day at a minimum; five a day is recommended. Fruits and vegetables contain many different antioxidant compounds, which are probably responsible for the anticancer effect of these foods. In addition, they offer many important vitamins and minerals, as well as numerous phytochemicals—lycopene (found in tomatoes and watermelon), quercetin (found in onions), ajoene (found in garlic), coumarins (found in citrus fruits), indoles (found in cruciferous vegetables), and many others—that are potent cancer fighters. In addition, increasing the amounts of fruits and vegetables in your diet will automatically increase the amount of fiber you get, and a high-fiber diet seems to greatly reduce the likelihood of colon cancer and may also help prevent breast, cervical, and lung cancer.

Reducing the amount of fat in your diet can also help reduce the risk of cancer. The average American gets about 40 percent of his or her daily calories from fat. Current guidelines recommend that no more than 30 percent of your calories come from fat, and many physicians believe that 20 percent should be the maximum.

As you lower the *amount* of fat in your diet, lower the least healthy *type* of fat as well. Whenever possible, substitute monounsaturated fats, such as olive oil and camola oil, for polyunsaturated and animal fats. (For more information about the different kinds of dietary fat, see the section on High Cholesterol.)

Plants to Fight Cancer

Many of the most effective drugs used today to fight cancer are based on compounds found naturally in plants. One plant in the vinca family, *Catharanthus roseus,* is the source of two drugs, vinblastine and vincristine, that are used to treat a number of different cancers. Drugs derived from mayapple roots are used in treating lymphomas, certain types of lung cancer, some types of leukemia, and other cancers. The drug tamoxifen, which is derived from substances found in the bark of the Pacific yew tree, is a highly effective treatment for ovarian cancer. Although these valuable anticancer drugs are derived from common plants, they are not herbal treatments. Most parts of trees in the yew family, for example, are poisonous. Drinking or consuming any sort of herbal product based on yew will not help cancer (or anything else) and could be extremely dangerous.

Careful studies have shown that garlic may contain potent anticancer compounds that could help stimulate the immune system and hinder the growth of cancer cells. In large-scale studies in Italy and China, for example, people who ate a lot of garlic over a lifetime were found to have fewer cases of stomach cancer.

Another plant that may well help prevent cancer is tea—black tea, green tea, and oolong tea (the kind served in Chinese restaurants). Tea contains catechins, substances that may block the development of some cancers. Green tea, brewed in the ordinary way, has the highest concentration of catechins; oolong is next, followed by black tea. So far, the only evidence for tea is successful tests on laboratory animals, not humans, but it is possible that drinking two or three cups a day could help keep you from getting cancer.

Cancer is one of the most dreaded diseases, so it's not surprising that over the years any number of irresponsible herbal practitioners have advocated quack remedies. A false cure first advocated in the 1920s is the so-called Hoxey remedy. This approach recommended "blood purification" based on a vegetarian diet emphasizing high-potassium foods, coffee enemas, and daily doses of an herbal mixture that combined red clover flowers with a mysterious mixture of other herbs. This medically worthless remedy, or variations on it, is still sometimes recommended by herbalists. The leaves and flowers of sweet violet or heartsease (viola) were used to treat breast and lung cancer in the 1930s, but they, too, were shown to be ineffective. More recently, laetrile (amygdalin), an extract made from apricot pits, has been advocated as a cancer cure. Laetrile, also sometimes called vitamin B_{15} or pangamic acid, was carefully studied by the National Cancer Institute, which declared it worthless in 1980. European mistletoe has been extensively studied for its possible role in treating cancer, but thus far, there have been no positive results. In fact, European mistletoe has been banned in Canada since 1991. Chaparral has also been studied as a possible anticancer drug, but to so little good effect that the Food and Drug Administration removed it from its list of herbs generally recognized as safe in 1968 and presently considers it unsafe for human consumption.

Herbalists sometimes recommend tea made from pau d'arco bark as a cancer treatment. Some evidence suggests that this herb contains some cancer-fighting compounds, but in human trials, the results were so insignificant and the side effects were so severe that the tests were abandoned. Recent studies by Japanese scientists suggest that suma, a root from the Amazon rain forest, may have some anticancer properties. The evidence so far is very inconclusive. Despite the claims for any herb, there is no way to successfully self-treat cancer.

Treating cancer can be a long and arduous process, but in many cases, the chances of a good outcome are high. Modern medicine can do a lot to relieve pain and reduce the unpleasant side effects of chemotherapy and radiation therapy. For more information, see the sections on Chemotherapy and Radiation Therapy.

❖ Candidiasis
See Yeast Infections.

❖ Canker Sores
See Mouth Sores.

❖ Carpal Tunnel Syndrome

Jobs that involve repetitive hand motions—typing or assembly-line work, for example—can lead to carpal tunnel syndrome: pain, tingling, and numbness in the thumb and forefinger area. The reason is that the bones that form your wrist (the carpals) are held together on the underside by a tough membrane to form a rigid tunnel. Tendons and the median nerve pass through this tunnel and into your hand. If the tendons are irritated by constantly performing the same hand motion, they swell and put painful pressure on the nerve.

The first step in treating carpal tunnel syndrome is to discover what is causing it. Since repetitive motions are the usual culprit, try changing the position of your hands (by using a wrist rest when typing, for example) and taking frequent short breaks. Wrist splints from the drugstore may help in severe cases. Nonsteroidal anti-inflammatory drugs such as aspirin and ibuprofen can help relieve the swelling.

Some physicians feel that a deficiency of vitamin B_6 is at the root of carpal tunnel syndrome. Vitamin B_6 is necessary for healthy nerve tissue, so adding it to your diet may help. Herbs that contain vitamin B_6 include alfalfa, burdock root, catnip leaves, dandelion leaves, fenugreek seeds, kelp, and red clover flowers. Vitamin B_6 is also found in bee pollen. Use caution, however: too much vitamin B_6 (more than 100 milligrams daily) can be toxic. Consult your doctor before adding supplements.

❖ Cataracts

As you grow older, or if you have diabetes, the clear lens of one or both of your eyes may develop a cataract, or cloudy area. Your vision deteriorates, often becoming progressively more blurred and distorted.

At one time, cataracts were a leading cause of blindness. Today, corrective eyeglasses can compensate for the problem in its early stages. Later on, safe, simple, outpatient surgery can substitute an artificial lens for the clouded natural lens. This surgery is the most common eye operation, and it is done more than a million times a year in the United States.

Solid evidence shows that eating a diet high in vitamin A, beta-carotenes, vitamin C, and vitamin E can help prevent cataracts. These antioxidant nutrients are found in many fresh fruits and vegetables. In addition, there is some evidence that the anthocyanosides found in dried blueberries (also called bilberries) can help prevent eye problems, including cataracts. However, the high concentration of this substance required can't be obtained simply by eating the berries or drinking a tea made from them. A commerical bilberry extract that claims to be high in anthocyanosides is available at health food stores. If you have or think you have a cataract or any other eye disease such as glaucoma, discuss the use of anthocyanosides with your doctor before trying it.

Other herbal remedies that have sometimes been suggested for cataracts include eyebright, yellow dock, and goldenseal. Don't be fooled by any claims. These herbs will not prevent, slow down, or cure cataracts. There is no herb or any other substance that can dissolve cataracts. Any such claims are unsubstantiated.

❖ Chemotherapy

Chemotherapy is the use of drugs to treat cancer. Anticancer drugs destroy cancer cells by preventing them from growing or multiplying at one or more stages in their life cycle. Because some drugs work better together than alone, chemotherapy often involves more than one drug. This is called combination chemotherapy. Chemotherapy is also sometimes used along with surgery or radiation treatments. Depending on the type of cancer and its stage of development, chemotherapy can be used to cure the cancer, keep it from spreading, slow its growth, kill cells that have spread (metastasized) to other parts of the body, and relieve cancer symptoms.

Chemotherapy can be a difficult experience. The biggest problem is generally side effects from the medications. Anticancer drugs are designed to kill fast-growing cancer cells. Unfortunately, they also can affect normal cells that grow rapidly, such as those in the digestive system, bone marrow, and hair follicles. The most common side effects of chemotherapy are nausea and vomiting, hair loss, and fatigue. Loss of appetite, diarrhea, constipation, sore mouth or throat, and changes in the taste of food are other possible side effects. Only about a third of cancer patients have side effects, however, and most side effects end when the treatment does.

Eating well during chemotherapy can help you cope better with the side effects of the treatment. If nausea and vomiting make eating difficult, your doctor can prescribe antiemetic drugs, which are usually very helpful. You can also help yourself with these eating tips from the National Cancer Institute:

- Eat small meals spread throughout the day.
- Drink liquids at least an hour before or after meals, instead of with your meals. This keeps you from feeling full too quickly at mealtime.
- Eat and drink slowly.
- Avoid sweet, fried, or fatty foods.
- Chew your food well for easier digestion.
- Drink cool, clear, unsweetened fruit juices.
- Suck on ice cubes made from plain water or frozen fruit juice, or try ice pops made from fruit juice without added sugar.
- If you are nauseous in the morning, eat dry toast, crackers, or dry cereal as soon as you wake up.

- Rest in a chair after eating. Don't lie flat for at least two hours after a meal.

Mouth sores are another side effect that can cause eating problems. Your doctor can prescribe pain-relieving medication to apply directly to the affected areas. Discuss the use of herbal remedies for mouth sores with your doctor before you try them.

Diarrhea is a common side effect of chemotherapy. Drink plenty of clear fluids such as water, apple juice, diluted fruit nectars, and weak tea (mild herbal teas such as peppermint and chamomile are good), but avoid milk and milk products, coffee, and alcohol. If you would like to try any herbal remedies for diarrhea, discuss them with your doctor first.

If any of your side effects are very severe or continue for a long time, be sure to call your doctor. You may need additional treatment to relieve the symptoms.

Chemotherapy is usually given in cycles that include rest periods to give your body a chance to regain its strength. Take advantage of the rest periods to eat a varied and nutritious diet. It's important to get enough calories and protein to keep your weight up and help your body repair itself.

Some medications, including over-the-counter drugs such as cold pills, can interfere with the beneficial effects of chemotherapy. So can many herbal remedies or large doses of vitamin and mineral supplements. Be sure to consult your doctor before taking any drugs, herbs, or supplements.

❖ Chronic Fatigue Syndrome

One of the most controversial illnesses of recent years, chronic fatigue syndrome (CFS) is sometimes called yuppie flu. Some doctors believe that it is caused by the Epstein Barr virus. Other doctors point out that a very large number of people have been infected with Epstein Barr virus but have no symptoms at all; these physicians often attribute CFS symptoms to stress or depression. The number of people reported to suffer from CFS is controversial too; estimates range from a hundred thousand to over a million current cases.

In general, CFS symptoms include severe fatigue, headaches, muscle and joint pain, tender lymph nodes, low-grade fever, sore throat, unrefreshing sleep, difficulty in concentrating, forgetfulness, and depression. There is no test for CFS, but the presence of severe fatigue along with four or more of the common symptoms is now considered diagnostic.

Since there is no proven cause of CFS, neither is there a proven treatment nor cure. Beware of potentially dangerous and fraudulent treatments that include injections with hydrogen peroxide (which can cause blood clots and trigger a stroke), high colonic enemas, bee pollen, and aloe vera juice (a powerful and dangerous laxative). Most doctors advise plenty of rest and a nutritious, varied diet with plenty of fresh fruits and vegetables. Some patients claim that eating yogurt with live acidophilus culture helps them feel better overall; others say that drinking fresh juice made from green leafy vegetables such as alfalfa increases their flagging energy levels. Some popular herbal remedies include teas made from pau d'arco bark, goldenseal, burdock root, or dandelion leaves. There is no evidence, however, that any of these herbs have any effect whatsoever on CFS symptoms.

❖ Cold Sores

The painful blisters of a cold sore on your lip are caused by the herpes simplex virus, type 1. Almost everyone gets infected by this very common virus in childhood. Most of the time, it remains dormant, but it can flare up into a cold sore if your immune system is weakened from illness, fever, stress, sunlight, or other causes.

Some evidence suggests that a diet high in the amino acid lysine and low in the amino acid arginine can help prevent cold sores. Lysine-rich foods such as brewer's yeast, milk, meat, and soybeans seem to block reproduction of the herpes virus, while arginine-rich foods such as chocolate, gelatin, and nuts seem to boost reproduction. If you have frequent outbreaks of cold sores, try avoiding arginine-rich foods and take 2,000 to 3,000 milligrams of supplemental lysine a day.

Once a cold sore has begun to develop, try treating the itching, tingling, and pain with plain petroleum jelly. You could also try applying tea tree oil or lavender oil to the blisters. In Europe, a cream containing the herb melissa (also called balm) is used to shorten the healing time of cold sores and decrease their recurrences. Since the cream is currently not available in the U.S., you could try applying a compress soaked in a strong infusion of balm to your cold sore several times a day. In severe cases, cold sores can be treated with the antiviral drug acyclovir.

Many physicians feel that cold sores can be prevented by protecting your lips against sun and wind. Frequent application of a lip balm that also contains a sunscreen will probably reduce the frequency of your cold sores.

❖ Colds

If you're a typical adult American, you're afflicted with the misery of a cold an average of three times a year. Your running nose, sneezing, sore throat, coughing, and overall malaise could be caused by one of some two hundred possible viruses. Although most colds go away in anywhere from three to seven days, you may be able to lessen the symptoms or cut short their duration with simple herbal remedies.

Echinacea, also sometimes called purple coneflower, is used by herbalists to stimulate your immune system and increase your body's resistance to infection. The usual recommendation is to take echinacea in tincture form (follow the package directions) at the first sign of a cold and to continue taking it while cold symptoms persist. Although scientists are still uncertain as to exactly how echinacea works, there is no doubt that it can be helpful. Astragalus root, a traditional Chinese herb, is sometimes suggested for fighting off a cold. The evidence for its effectiveness is slim to nonexistent.

If you have a running nose, you need to compensate for all the mucus your body is discharging by drinking plenty of liquids. Drinking liquids also helps keep the mucus membranes lining your respiratory tract moist, making them less hospitable to the cold virus. Most doctors suggest six to eight glasses of preferably warm liquid a day. Avoid sweetened beverages and fruit juices in favor of plain water, weak tea, and mild herbal teas, such as peppermint, linden flowers, red raspberry leaves, or chamomile. Many people find that ginger root tea helps temporarily relieve their cold symptoms, especially upper respiratory congestion.

Eating lots of garlic and onions may help boost your immune system and fight off the cold virus. Eating hot chili peppers may also help fight the virus, and this will definitely help clear your congested nose and sinuses.

The belief that vitamin C prevents or cures colds is widely accepted, but there's actually little evidence to prove it. Even so, many cold sufferers swear that taking anywhere from 500 to 1,000 milligrams of supplemental vitamin C a day reduces the frequency of their colds, shortens the duration of any colds they do get, and reduces the symptoms. Let the vitamin C buyer beware: Allegedly organic vitamin C tablets derived from rose hips are no different from any other sort of vitamin C tablet. Don't waste your money on fraudulent claims of purity.

Colds almost always go away on their own. Sometimes, however, a cold can lead to an ear infection, sinusitis, bronchitis, or some other infection. See your doctor if your cold symptoms get markedly worse after a few days, if you're still not feeling better after ten days, or if you develop an earache, facial pain, high temperature, or bad cough. Also see your doctor if the symptoms include a sore throat with a high fever, especially where a child is concerned. The problem could be strep throat.

See also Bronchitis; Coughs; Influenza; Sore Throat.

❖ Colic

Excessive crying in babies, also known as colic, can be very distressing and exhausting for both the baby and the parents. Colic usually begins when the baby is only a few weeks old. Fortunately, it almost always ends naturally by the time the baby is six months old. Colic occurs in 15 percent or more of all newborns. It doesn't mean that your baby is unhealthy or sick, and it doesn't occur because of anything you do or don't do.

Colicky babies may seem to be having digestive troubles, because they often eat poorly, pull their legs up as if they have a stomachache, have gas, and seem to be in pain. The gas is probably from all the air the baby swallows from crying so much. Proper burping after feeding may help relieve some of the gas. Also, try switching to a nipple with a smaller hole or offering smaller, more frequent feedings if your baby usually sucks quickly and completes a bottle feeding in less than twenty minutes. Nobody really knows what causes colic, although dietary factors may be at work.

Traditional herbal remedies for gas pains and colic in babies include chamomile flowers, fennel seeds, and lavender flowers. Try making these herbs, singly or in combination, into strong teas and adding five to ten drops to the baby's bottle at each feeding. Nursing women can try drinking a cup of chamomile tea before breast-feeding.

❖ Colitis
See Irritable Bowel Syndrome.

❖ Congestive Heart Failure

Congestive heart failure occurs when your heart is weakened by disease or by a faulty valve and can no longer pump blood efficiently through your body. If the left side of your heart is affected, it will not pump blood to your lungs well, and you will probably feel breathless. If the right side of your heart is affected, it will not pump blood to the rest of your body very well. You may feel tired, and fluid will probably start to accumulate in the lower part of your body, especially your feet, ankles, and legs (this condition is called edema). If both sides of your heart are affected, a combination of the symptoms described above is likely.

Heart failure is a serious problem that can be successfully treated with medications that help your heart beat better and thin your blood to avoid dangerous blood clots. You may also need to take diuretics and sharply reduce your salt intake to prevent fluid retention. Eliminating table salt from the diet is not enough. Many processed foods, baked goods, and some over-the-counter medications also contain salt or sodium. Monosodium glutamate (MSG), for example, is often added to processed foods; baking soda contains sodium, too. Many nonprescription medications for heartburn contain sodium bicarbonate. Read all labels carefully and do everything you can to avoid consuming hidden salt.

Some people feel that traditional diuretic herbs, such as lovage, chicory, and bearberry (uva ursi), are natural substances and thus are somehow better than prescribed diuretics. This misconception could prove very dangerous when it comes to treating congestive heart failure. These herbs are neither very effective nor very predictable in their effects and potencies, especially if you take them in combination with prescription drugs. If your doctor prescribes a diuretic drug, take it as directed. If you wish to use any herbal remedies, discuss them with your doctor first.

If you have congestive heart failure, avoid any herbal medication containing licorice root. It can cause fluid retention and edema. Also avoid ephedra (also called ma huang), goldenseal, and yohimbe if you have congestive heart failure.

One of the earliest successful treatments for congestive heart failure was digitalis, the dried leaves of the purple foxglove plant. Foxglove is a popular garden flower, but do not attempt to treat congestive heart failure on your own with homemade digitalis.

Extracts containing hawthorn flowers and berries are a traditional European herbal remedy for various heart problems. The active ingredients in hawthorn are being studied for their possible beneficial effects on the heart, but right now, commercial remedies containing hawthorn are not available in the United States. Traditional herbal medicine classifies some herbs as heart tonics. These include lobelia, skullcap, lily of the valley, motherwort, and ginseng. Congestive heart failure is a serious condition, however, and one that responds well to standard drug therapy. Do not attempt to treat congestive heart failure with herbal medicine.

❖ Constipation

Although many people believe that a daily bowel movement is essential to good health, the normal frequency of bowel movements varies widely from person to person. Some have several movements a day, while others may defecate as infrequently as three times a week. You are constipated or irregular only if you have fewer movements than usual, or if the stool is hard, dry, and difficult to pass.

Traditional herbal practitioners and naturopaths place tremendous emphasis on bowel regularity, believing that a wide range of minor ailments—from acne to yeast infections—are caused by constipation or colon sluggishness and that they can be relieved by cleansing the colon. There is very little evidence to back up recommendations for the frequent use of laxatives and enemas, however. These treatments are almost always unnecessary and can be quite unpleasant, or even dangerous.

For almost everyone, constipation is a result of a diet that has too little fiber or not enough liquids. Lack of exercise and failure to respond to the urge to defecate can also contribute to constipation. Some prescription and over-the-counter drugs can cause constipation, including antacids, iron pills, and calcium supplements. If you think a prescription drug is causing your constipation, and increasing the amount of fiber and liquid you consume doesn't help, discuss the problem with your doctor.

If you eat a lot of fiber (at least 30 grams a day) and drink plenty of liquids (six to eight glasses a day), you are unlikely to become constipated. If you do, try eating a handful of dried prunes, apricots, or figs, or a large glass of prune juice. These fruits contain isatin, a natural laxative. You should get results within twenty-four hours.

Herbalists often recommend stimulant herbs such as cascara sagrada bark, buckthorn bark, and senna to treat constipation. These herbs contain anthraquinones, which cause your lower intestine to absorb less water from the stool. Cascara and senna are ingredients in some over-the-counter remedies for constipation; buckthorn is botanically very similar to cascara. All three are gentle stimulants. Cascara and buckthorn are usually taken in the form of liquid extracts; just 1/2 teaspoon is usually effective. Senna is usually taken as an extract, syrup, or tablets. The usual dosage is 1/2 teaspoon for the liquid forms or 1 or 2 tablets. These remedies may all cause intestinal griping and diarrhea. Since they can be passed on through breast milk, they should be avoided by nursing women.

Two stimulant herbs should be avoided: rhubarb and aloe. Rhubarb is quite potent and can cause severe intestinal griping. Aloe (not to be confused with fresh aloe vera gel) is even more potent and uncomfortable. Both ingredients are found in a popular European herbal preparation called Swedish bitters.

The traditional Chinese herb fo-ti does have a mild laxative effect, but many traditional European or North American herbs, including yellow dock, dandelion root, and licorice root, are basically worthless, despite their reputations.

Doctors generally discourage the use of stimulant laxatives, even natural ones. They can cause your intestines to become lazy, so that you become dependent on the laxative to move your bowels. Laxatives can interfere with medications, and can cause foods to move through your intestines too rapidly for the nutrients to be absorbed by your body.

When a laxative is necessary, physicians generally recommend the bulk-forming kind because these most naturally resemble the way the body works. Bulk-forming laxatives add bulk and water to your stools so that they can pass through the intestines more easily. Psyllium seed husks, also called plantago seed, is the ingredient found in over-the-counter bulk laxatives such as Metamucil. These laxatives should be taken with a full glass of water, juice, or other fluid. Results usually occur in twelve to twenty-four hours, but may take longer for some people.

❖ Contact Dermatitis

Contact dermatitis is any swelling, itchiness, blistering, flaking, or redness of the skin due to contact with an irritating substance. Sunburn, poison ivy, and nickel allergy are common forms of contact dermatitis. Soaps, detergents, and shampoos can also cause this condition.

Dermatitis often clears up on its own when contact with the offending substance is eliminated. Wearing latex gloves while you wash dishes, for example, usually solves the problem of dishpan hands. The irritant nickel is commonly found in costume jewelry and in gold jewelry that contains less than 24 karats.

To relieve the symptoms of contact dermatitis, try a compress soaked in witch hazel. The tannin in the witch hazel has an astringent effect that temporarily relieves itching and helps dry up blisters. Distilled witch hazel is made from twigs and has virtually no tannins. Purchase a nondistilled extract of witch hazel leaves from a well-stocked health food store.

See also Eczema; Poison Ivy; Psoriasis; Sunburn.

❖ Coughs

The persistent coughing that accompanies bronchitis or a cold is one of the most annoying of symptoms. It can keep you—and everyone within earshot of you—from getting any rest. Even more annoying is that the cough may continue for weeks after the original illness is over. Perhaps because coughing is so common and so aggravating, scores of herbs have been recommended as remedies for it over the centuries. Some traditional herbal remedies for coughing are, in fact, helpful. Most fall into two categories: demulcent antitussive (cough suppressants) and expectorants.

The most effective herbal cough suppressants are made from herbs that contain mucilage. The mucilage coats the mucous membranes of your throat, which reduces irritation in the area and thus blocks your urge to cough. Coltsfoot, an herb that has been popular as an herbal cough remedy for centuries, contains a high level of mucilage. It also contains high levels of toxic alkaloids, however, and for that reason should not be used for coughs or anything else. Slippery elm bark, a remedy popular with Native Americans and early settlers, is safe and helpful. It can be taken as a tea, but it is most effective when taken in lozenge form, which can be found in health food stores. Tea made from marshmallow root is helpful. Steep 1 or 2 teaspoonfuls in 1 cup of boiling water and sip throughout the day. Plantain leaves (plantago) is another safe and popular cough remedy. Make a tea using 3 to 4 teaspoons of leaves to 1 cup boiling water. Drink no more than two cups daily. Mullein flowers have a fairly low mucilage content compared to the herbs above, but they can still be helpful. Make them into a tea using 3 to 4 teaspoons to 1 cup boiling water. You can safely drink 3 to 4 cups a day. Iceland moss (really a lichen) is very high in mucilage. Make it into a strong tea, using 2 to 3 teaspoonfuls to 1 cup boiling water. Drink no more than 3 cups a day. Iceland moss is high in lead. Do not give it to children; adults should not use it for more than a week.

Expectorants help thin the mucus and make it easier to cough it up. Several herbs make effective expectorants. One of the best-known and most pleasant-tasting is made from the leaves and flowers of horehound. Horehound was used in some over-the-counter cough medicines until 1989, when it was banned by the Food and Drug Administration. The reason was that it had not been shown to be effective, although the FDA does still consider horehound to be generally recognized as safe. Horehound is approved for use in Germany. To make horehound tea, steep 2 to 3 teaspoonfuls in 2 cups boiling water; drink no more than 5 cups a day. Horehound lozenges are readily available at health food stores. Senega snakeroot, another Native American remedy, is often very helpful for thinning mucus. Make it into a strong tea, using just a pinch of ground, dried root in 1 cup of boiling water. Drink no more than 5 cups a day; any more than that could cause stomach upset and diarrhea.

Teas made from thyme, anise seeds, fennel seeds, and peppermint leaves act as mild expectorants. Primula flowers and root are popular in Europe but are difficult to find in the United States. Licorice root tea is also effective, but should be avoided by people with high blood pressure or heart problems, since it can cause fluid retention. Lobelia (also called Indian tobacco) is another traditional expectorant herb that is still recommended by some herbalists. It contains toxic alkaloids, however, and should not be used.

Coughing can sometimes indicate a more serious problem. If you start coughing but don't have an upper respiratory infection, such as a cold, you might have lung cancer. If a bad cough doesn't improve after a few days or go away after a couple of weeks, or if you cough up blood or bloody phlegm, see your doctor. If you have chronic bronchitis, asthma, heart disease, or any other chronic condition, see your doctor before using any herbal remedy for coughing.

See also Bronchitis; Colds; Influenza.

❖ Cuts, Scrapes, and Wounds

Most minor cuts and scrapes will heal up by themselves within a week or so, leaving no scar. They generally require no treatment beyond basic first aid. Some herbs, however, can help speed up the healing process, prevent infection, and relieve pain.

Applying fresh aloe vera gel to a cut or scrape can be very helpful. Aloe vera is known to have antibacterial properties that can help prevent infection. Research indicates that it may also block pain-producing substances in the body and promote healing. The beneficial effect of aloe vera is available only when it is used in the fresh form or in a stabilized gel. Many commercial creams and ointments contain aloe vera that has been reconstituted or made from an extract. These products are not particularly effective.

Calendula is a traditional and effective herbal remedy for healing wounds. Apply calendula cream or ointment sparingly to the affected area. Tea tree oil has some antiseptic and anesthetic effect on wounds, too.

Arnica is often used on bruises, but do not apply it to broken skin. Comfrey is another traditional herbal remedy that does offer some minor benefits. These are significantly offset, however, by the toxic alkaloids this herb also contains. Do not use comfrey on wounds, and never take it internally.

Herbal remedies are sometimes suggested for wounds that are slow to heal. Slow healing is often an indication of a more serious underlying problem, such as diabetes. If you have a wound that isn't healing well, don't attempt to treat it yourself. See your doctor.

❖ Cystitis
See Urinary Tract Infections.

❖ Dandruff

Unsightly dandruff, or flaking of the scalp, occurs when your body starts to replace the skin cells of your scalp at a rate faster than usual. The dead skin cells slough off and appear as white flakes. Although dandruff is a problem, in varying degrees of severity, for about 35 percent of all Americans, no one really knows what causes the skin cells to turn over so rapidly. Doctors do know, however, that dandruff usually begins in puberty, gets worse in young adults, and levels off or even disappears by middle age. It's not a disease and there is no cure. It's not caused by washing your hair too often, but washing your hair daily with a gentle shampoo often helps mild cases.

Numerous herbal or folk remedies exist for dandruff, and some may actually help. One old folk treatment is to rub a mixture of cider vinegar and water into your scalp. Let it stay for fifteen minutes, then rinse it off. Instead of the vinegar treatment, you could try witch hazel or strong teas made from chamomile, sage, or rosemary. Jojoba oil can be very effective, especially in mild cases. Shampoos containing jojoba oil can be found in any drugstore or health food store.

❖ Depression

Feeling mildly down or blue once in a while for a few hours, or even several days, is very common—so common that it's considered completely normal. For this sort of mild depression, many doctors suggest a simple remedy: a cup of coffee. Caffeine is a mild stimulant that may temporarily elevate your mood. Other herbs that contain caffeine in lesser amounts include tea, guarana, and maté.

Other herbs may also lift your spirits as well. A popular European herbal remedy for depression is a tea made from the leaves and flowers of St. John's wort. Drink no more than 3 cups a day. If you take St. John's wort for long periods, it may cause your skin to become sensitive to sunlight. If this occurs, stop using the herb until the sensitivity goes away; take it less often, or in smaller doses, if you resume use. Interestingly, St. John's wort has an effect that's similar to monoamine oxidase (MAO) inhibitors, a type of drug often prescribed for serious depression. People taking prescription MAO inhibitors should avoid eating aged, fermented, and pickled foods, so it may be a good idea to avoid these foods when taking St. John's wort. Numerous other herbs, generally in tea form, are said to help relieve mild depression. These include ginger, sage, peppermint, borage, lemon balm, and skullcap. Of these, lemon balm is said to be particularly effective.

Hops is sometimes used as an herbal aid for insomnia. If your insomnia is related to feeling depressed, however, do not use hops. This herb has a mildly depressive effect and could make you feel worse.

The amino acid L-tryptophan, while not an herb, is often recommended as an antidepressive and sedative. Since 1989, however, when it was linked to twenty-seven deaths and over 5,000 cases of serious illness, L-tryptophan has been banned by the Food and Drug Administration.

Depressive disorders, unlike mild depression or a passing feeling of sadness, won't respond to home herbal remedies. Without medical treatment, the condition can last for weeks, months, or years. According to the National Institute for Mental Health, in any six-month period, nine million American adults suffer from a depressive illness. If you feel deeply depressed for more than a week, talk about it with your doctor or someone else you can trust. Depression can sometimes follow a distressing emotional event, such as divorce or a death in the family, but often it just happens, as any other illness does.

❖ Dermatitis
See Eczema.

❖ Diabetes

An estimated thirteen to fourteen million people in the United States have diabetes, making it one of the country's biggest health problems. Diabetes is the seventh leading cause of death in the United States and the single leading cause of kidney disease; it's also a leading cause of blindness. More than 250,000 Americans die each year from causes directly related to this disease. Diabetics also have double the risk of the general population for heart attack and stroke.

There are two types of diabetes. Insulin-dependent diabetes (type I) affects only about 5 to 10 percent of people with the disease and first occurs predominantly in children. Because type I diabetes is a serious and complex illness that requires careful treatment, herbal remedies are not recommended, and there is no room to discuss it in this book.

The majority of people with diabetes—between 90 and 95 percent—have noninsulin dependent (type II) diabetes (also called adult-onset diabetes). This form of diabetes usually begins in adults over age forty, and is most common after age fifty-five. Nearly half the people who have noninsulin dependent diabetes don't know it because the symptoms develop gradually and are hard to identify at first. Diabetes often has some clear warning signs. See your doctor at once if you have any of these symptoms:

- Frequent urination
- Constant feeling of thirst
- Fatigue
- Slow healing of skin, gums, and urinary tract infections
- Sudden weight loss
- Blurred vision

If you have type II diabetes, your pancreas usually produces the normal amount of insulin you need to help your cells use the glucose (digested sugar) in your blood for energy. Instead, for unknown reasons, your cells have become insensitive to insulin, a condition called insulin resistance. In some cases, people who are insulin-resistant compensate for it by producing even more insulin in the pancreas. Most people, however, can't produce enough additional insulin to overcome the resistance. As a result, glucose builds up in the blood and causes the symptoms of diabetes.

Obese people are at greatest risk for developing type II diabetes. Physicians estimate that 60 to 90 percent of the people with this type of diabetes are overweight. There are two other major risk factors: having a parent with type II diabetes and being a member of certain minority groups. Among African-Americans, type II diabetes occurs 1.5 times more often than among white Americans; among Hispanics and Orientals, it occurs more than twice as often.

Noninsulin-dependent diabetes can be controlled by losing weight, eating an appropriate diet, exercising regularly, and taking medication as prescribed by your doctor. (Only about a third of all type II diabetics need to inject insulin.) If you smoke and have diabetes, stop. Diabetic smokers run a much, much greater risk of heart attack and stroke. Diabetics should also avoid alcohol. The condition already places the liver and pancreas under stress, and drinking alcohol can damage these organs. The empty calories of alcohol can also make controlling your blood glucose more difficult.

Many diabetics find that their symptoms begin to improve or even go away completely if they lose weight, even a little. In fact, if you are obese and have diabetes, losing only ten pounds can help you reduce your level of insulin resistance. The sooner you lose the weight, the better. Studies show that the longer you have diabetes, the less of an effect losing weight will have.

The goal of diabetes treatment is to keep your blood glucose within normal range and to prevent long-term complications such as heart disease, kidney disease, blindness, and blood vessel problems. There's no one diabetic diet. In general, a healthy diet that is high in fiber, low in fat, low in sodium, and includes a variety of foods will help. Your doctor can advise you on how to modify your diet.

The mineral chromium is a component of glucose tolerance factor (GTF), a substance your body produces that works with insulin to help your cells use glucose. The recommended daily allowance of chromium is between 50 and 200 micrograms. Some diabetics find that eating foods high in chromium helps them control their blood glucose. Good dietary sources of chromium are brewer's yeast, whole grain breads and cereals (especially buckwheat and barley), molasses, cheese, nuts, orange juice, and broccoli. When eaten as part of a well-balanced diet, these foods could help your diabetes. Some diabetics take supplements containing chromium picolinate instead. However, too much chromium can actually inhibit the effectiveness of insulin. Also, if you take diabetes medication, you may need to adjust the dosage if you add chromium to your diet. Discuss increasing your chromium intake with your doctor first.

Recent research suggests that the spices cinnamon, turmeric, bay leaves, and cloves may help your body use insulin more effectively. Cinnamon may be especially helpful. Try sprinkling a little on your food.

Proponents of herbal treatments have sometimes suggested huckleberry leaf tea, huckleberries, sarsaparilla, fenugreek seeds, blue-green algae, burdock root, juniper berries, dandelion root, goldenseal, evening primrose oil, uva ursi, angelica, and ginseng as ways to treat diabetes. These herbs are said to either naturally increase your body's production of insulin or normalize blood sugar levels. Recent research suggests that fenugreek seeds might increase sensitivity to insulin, but herbal treatments should never be used in place of losing weight, diet, exercise, and medicine for treating diabetes. There is no antidiabetes herb. If you use or are thinking of using an herbal treatment for diabetes, discuss it with your doctor.

Patients who take charge of their diabetes and work with their doctor to keep it under control have a good chance of leading normal lives and avoiding complications. For more information on living well with diabetes, contact:

American Diabetes Association
1660 Duke Street
Alexandria, VA 22314-3447
800/232-3472

❖ Dialysis

Your kidneys remove waste products from your blood and regulate the balance of water and chemicals in your body. When your kidneys no longer function properly—either temporarily or permanently—their work must be done artificially by dialysis. There are two kinds of dialysis: peritoneal dialysis and hemodialysis. In peritoneal dialysis, a special fluid flows through a tube inserted into your abdomen and fills up the peritoneal space. Waste products and excess water from your blood enter the fluid, which then drains out again through another tube. Peritoneal dialysis is a continuous process that can take several hours. Hemodialysis uses a kidney machine to remove wastes and excess water directly from your blood. Blood passes from a tube in an artery of your arm or leg into the machine, and then is sent back through another tube into a vein. The process generally takes several hours, three times a week. Peritoneal dialysis and hemodialysis can often be performed at home without medical assistance, but many people who need hemodialysis go to special centers equipped with kidney machines and specially trained medical personnel.

Diet is extremely important for dialysis patients. In general, dialysis patients need to be very careful about the amounts of protein, potassium, sodium, and phosphorus they consume. They also need to be sure they are getting enough calories, vitamins, and minerals, but not too much fluid. To help you deal with the complexities of dialysis, your doctor will probably refer you to a specially trained renal (kidney) dietitian. By working with the dietitian and paying close attention to diet, your dialysis can go much more smoothly.

Maintaining the right level of potassium, a mineral found naturally in many foods, is vital for dialysis patients, because the dialysis process removes potassium from the body. Balance is important because both high *and* low levels of potassium are dangerous to your heart, and high levels can even lead to death. Potassium is found in large amounts in dried fruits, dried beans and peas, nuts, meat, milk, fruits, and vegetables. Salt substitutes are another rich source. Many common herbs and other natural remedies also contain potassium. If you are on dialysis, avoid alfalfa, bee pollen, blue cohosh, chamomile, dandelion, echinazea, kelp, nettle, white oak bark, yarrow, and yellow dock. Discuss using any herbs or other remedies with your doctor before you try them.

Dialysis treatment washes some water-soluble vitamins from your body. Patients on hemodialysis often develop a type of anemia due to a lack of vitamin E. Also, the limited diet you must follow could mean that you don't get enough vitamins and minerals. Discuss taking supplements with your doctor, however, since too much of certain vitamins may be harmful.

❖ Diarrhea

Diarrhea—the frequent passing of loose, watery stools—is your body's way of getting rid of germs or an offending food. Fortunately, in adults this common but usually minor ailment generally goes away within a couple of days. Taking some simple self-help measures can relieve the symptoms and help you feel better faster. However, diarrhea in infants, children, chronically ill people, and the elderly can be very serious. Call your doctor.

Instead of trying to stop the diarrhea, doctors generally suggest that you just try to replace the fluids your body loses. Most doctors recommend drinking lots of clear fluids and diluted fruit juices. Water is always good, as are old stand-bys such as flat ginger ale, chicken broth, weak tea, and mild peppermint or chamomile tea. Some people find that sports drinks are helpful.

Dried (not fresh) blueberries are a traditional European remedy for diarrhea that can help relieve symptoms. Soak a teaspoonful or so of the berries in 1 cup boiling water until the berries are softened, about five minutes. Drink the liquid and then eat the berries. Repeat three to seven times daily. The tannins and pectin in the blueberries are what make this remedy effective. Teas made from blackberry, raspberry, or blueberry leaves, from blackberry root, and from wood betony are helpful because they, too, are high in tannin. Use 1 to 2 teaspoons of leaves to 1 cup boiling water. Let steep for ten to fifteen minutes before drinking. If you use blackberry root, let it steep for twenty minutes.

As soon as you feel like eating again, try having something that is thick, starchy, and not too sweet. It's usually best to eat several small meals spread throughout the day rather than one or two big meals. Once you're on the mend, eating some live-culture yogurt or taking acidophilus tablets can help restore the balance of good bacteria in your digestive tract.

Sometimes diarrhea is caused by the artificial sweeteners sorbitol or mannitol, which are often used in dietetic baked goods, candies, and chewing gum. Sorbitol is also found naturally in apple juice, pear juice, and grape juice. Another cause of diarrhea could be nonprescription liquid antacids containing magnesium hydroxide. High doses of vitamin C can cause diarrhea. If you take supplemental vitamin C, try cutting back. Prescription antibiotics can cause diarrhea because they also kill the useful bacteria in your digestive tract. If you think an antibiotic is causing your diarrhea, try eating some live-culture yogurt or taking acidophilus tablets. If the diarrhea persists, discuss a change of medication with you doctor.

Diarrhea that doesn't go away in a few day or that recurs often can be a sign of a more serious problem. See your doctor without delay.

See also Irritable Bowel Syndrome.

❖ Dry Skin

If the air that surrounds you is very dry, it could lead to itchy, dry skin. Dry skin is often a winter problem, since heat from radiators dries the air. Turning down the heat and adding moisture back to the air by using a humidifier can help quite a bit at home, but you can't stay at home all day. Instead, you'll have to add moisture back to the skin. An amazing array of moisturizers is available at any drugstore, ranging from plain, inexpensive petroleum jelly to outrageously priced formulas from cosmetic manufacturers. Moisturizers that contain aloe are often very effective and have a pleasant aroma. If you have problems with perfumes and other ingredients, look for unscented or hypoallergenic products.

The itchiness of dry skin can be soothed by an oatmeal bath. You can purchase colloidal oatmeal (Aveeno brand) at the drugstore, or make it yourself by grinding ordinary rolled oats in a food processor until they are a fine powder. Put 2 cups into a tub of lukewarm water and soak for twenty minutes or so.

See also Eczema; Psoriasis.

❖ Ear Infections

Painful infections of the middle ear (otitis media) are very common among young children. Generally, an infection occurs because the child's short eustachian tubes, which drain fluid from the middle ear, are blocked by swelling from a cold or allergies. The usual medical treatment for middle ear infections is antibiotics to clear up the infection and acetaminophen (Tylenol) to relieve the pain. Some parents are very concerned about the effects antibiotics might have on their children. Ear infections are very painful, however, and there is a real risk of serious and permanent damage to the child's hearing if the infection is not treated. The risks of antibiotic treatment are far outweighed by the benefits.

Ignore recommendations to put a few drops of herbal oil into the ear canal. Middle ear infections affect the eardrum, sometimes making it bulge or even break. If the eardrum has broken, the oil could make the infection considerably worse. Only use eardrops prescribed by your doctor.

If your child has frequent ear infections, you could try giving him or her a few drops of echinacea tincture every day. This herb may help the child ward off future infections by stimulating the immune system.

Breast-fed babies usually have fewer ear infections, since they receive antibodies to respiratory infections from their mothers. If you're considering breast-feeding, this is another good reason to do so. If you bottle-feed, always make sure the baby's head is elevated while he drinks; otherwise, fluid can get into his eustachian tubes and cause discomfort and an infection. When a child has an ear infection, elevate the head at night to help fluid drain from the eustachian tubes.

Because swallowing helps keep the eustachian tubes open, small, frequent sips of liquid can help relieve discomfort. Breathing clean, moist air also helps. Use a humidifier and avoid wood smoke and cigarette smoke.

❖ Eating Disorders
See Anorexia Nervosa.

❖ Eczema

Eczema—patches of swollen, red, flaky, itchy, or blistered skin—is a very common condition. In many cases, it's caused by contact with an irritating substance, such as harsh soaps or chemicals. Stop the contact by wearing rubber gloves to do the dishes, for example, and the eczema goes away. Eczema can also be an allergic reaction, often to something you have eaten. Be on guard for any foods that make your eczema flare up, and avoid them.

Sometimes a compress soaked in witch hazel relieves the itching and weeping of eczema. This only works if the witch hazel still has its natural tannins. Distilled witch hazel is made from twigs and has virtually no tannins. You can usually purchase a nondistilled extract of witch hazel leaves at a well-stocked health food store. Another good way to relieve eczema symptoms is with a milk compress. Soak a gauze square or washcloth in ice-cold milk and hold it against the affected area for a few minutes; repeat twice more. Use this treatment several times a day.

Creams and ointments made with chickweed, stinging nettle, heartsease, calendula, and yellow dock have all been recommended by herbalists for eczema. These may provide some minor relief, but it's probably due to the soothing effect of the cream or ointment base, not the herbs. Chickweed, for example, contains very little in the way of active compounds, and the few it does have of are no use for eczema. There's also little evidence that drinking red clover tea can help.

Evening primrose oil, black currant oil, borage seed oil, and linseed oil are sometimes suggested as treatments for eczema. These oils contain gamma-linolenic acid (GLA), a fatty acid your body needs to make hormonelike substances called prostaglandins. It is thought that a deficiency of prostaglandins is a cause of many ailments, including eczema. However, there is no evidence that supports this. Taking capsules of any of these oils is unlikely to help your eczema.

The itchiness of eczema can be soothed by an oatmeal bath. You can purchase colloidal oatmeal (Aveeno brand) at the drugstore, or make it yourself by grinding ordinary rolled oats to a fine powder in a food processor. Add 2 cups to a tub of lukewarm water and soak for twenty minutes or so.

See also Contact Dermatitis; Psoriasis.

❖ Edema

See Congestive Heart Failure.

❖ Epilepsy

The human brain contains about twelve billion nerve cells, which communicate with each other and the rest of the body via electrical impulses. Epilepsy is the name given to disturbed electrical activity in the brain. The brain cells overload, and the result is a seizure—a temporary loss of consciousness often in association with motor activity. Two million Americans—one in every hundred—have epilepsy.

A great deal of herbal folklore, all of it specious, has grown up around epilepsy. Herbal remedies based on linden flowers, skullcap, passion flower, lobelia, sarsaparilla, black pepper, and brewer's yeast have all proven completely ineffective. Epileptics should avoid sage, also called dan shen in traditional Chinese medicine; it contains thujone, which in large quantities could trigger a seizure.

The amino acids L-glutamine, L-glycine, and L-threonine are sometimes recommended by practitioners of alternative medicine as natural compounds for controlling epilepsy. There is no evidence that they are effective. Large doses of single amino acids are unlikely to have any desired effect and are potentially toxic. The Food and Drug Administration does not consider single amino acids to be generally recognized as safe. Do not substitute amino acids for your usual epilepsy medication.

The artificial sweetener aspartame (NutraSweet) has sometimes been blamed for an increase in seizures among epileptics. Careful investigation has not yielded any data to support this claim.

❖ Eye Problems

Minor eye irritations and strains occur all the time. Looking at a computer monitor for long periods of time, reading in poor light, air pollution, cigarette or wood smoke, pollen allergies, airborne irritants, and many other causes can result in eyes that are tired, red-rimmed, bloodshot, watery, or itchy.

Eyebright is the herb most commonly recommended for minor eye irritations. This European herb bears spotted or striped flowers that have some resemblance to bloodshot eyes. For that reason, it has been used for centuries as an eye treatment, even though there is no evidence that it does any good. Herbalists sometimes suggest swallowing eyebright capsules or drinking eyebright tea, but more commonly, they recommend eyebright eyewash. If you wish to try eyebright capsules or tea, be certain that you are buying European eyebright (*Euphrasis*) and not any other herb.

Other herbs said to be helpful for eye irritation include goldenseal, yellow dock, red raspberry leaves, horsetail, elder leaves, chamomile, and hyssop. The recommendation usually is to make a tea from the herb and then use it as an eyewash. However, putting any sort of herbal eyewash, homemade or purchased, that isn't sterile into your eyes is dangerous. Herbal eyewashes won't help your irritated eyes and they could cause infection.

A cool compress made from a clean washcloth soaked in cold eyebright, chamomile, or other mild herbal tea (or plain cold water) can help soothe red, tired eyes. Lie down, place the compress on your closed eyes, and rest for ten minutes; repeat if necessary. Some people find a warm compress more soothing.

You can avoid eyestrain when working at a computer by using incandescent, not fluorescent, bulbs in nearby light fixtures and desk lamps. You could also try adjusting the brightness control on your monitor downward. Most people make their screen far too bright. As the natural light in your work area changes over the course of the day, readjust the brightness level. Take a ten-minute break every two hours.

Conjunctivitis (also called pinkeye), an inflammation of the membrane that lines your eyelids and the white of your eye, is a common ailment. It is usually caused by an infection or by allergies. Conjunctivitis from an infection should not be self-treated. See your doctor. If the conjunctivitis is caused by an allergy, try to avoid the allergen. It may be easier to avoid some allergens, such as cigarette smoke, but avoiding others, such as pollen, can be more difficult. Talk to your doctor about antihistamines.

See also Cataracts; Glaucoma; Sties.

❖ Fatigue

For most people, being tired all the time is such a common feeling that they accept it as normal. While it is natural to feel tired when you're under a lot of stress or not getting enough sleep, it's also possible that poor nutrition is contributing to the problem. Take a good look at your eating habits and make some positive changes. If you smoke, stop. If you drink alcohol, give it up or cut back. Smoking and drinking rob your body of nutrients.

Beverages containing caffeine, including coffee, tea, colas, guarana, and maté, all act as stimulants and can help temporarily relieve fatigue. For deep-seated, constant fatigue, traditional herbal remedies abound. Traditional Chinese herbal medicine often treats fatigue or lack of energy with ginseng, taken as a tea or in capsules containing powdered root; dong quai is also sometimes recommended. A traditional South American remedy is gotu kola tea. The traditional European recommendation is rosemary tea. Other herbal remedies include yellow dock, Iceland moss, and bee pollen.

Fatigue can be a warning sign that an illness such as a cold or flu is coming; if you suspect this, try taking some echinacea drops to help ward off illness. Fatigue can also be a symptom of diabetes, anemia, or chronic fatigue syndrome. See your doctor if you are severely fatigued for more than a few days for no obvious reason.

❖ Fever

Fever is a symptom of an illness or infection. Fever can be a normal, even helpful, response to the problem and will go away as you get better. If the fever is making you uncomfortable, most doctors suggest taking acetaminophen (Tylenol) to help bring it down.

Herbal remedies for fever abound. Willow bark tea is a traditional treatment, but as discussed in the section on arthritis, it is very bitter and unlikely to be very helpful unless you drink more than a gallon of it. Boneset tea is a traditional Native American treatment for fevers; it is even less effective than willow bark tea and tastes considerably worse. Feverfew, despite its name, is ineffective against fevers.

Teas made from chamomile, peppermint, red clover flowers, vervain, catnip, lemon balm, and other mild-tasting herbs are all often recommended as ways to reduce fever. Although they are ineffective for that purpose, they still may be helpful. Since you should drink plenty of liquids while you have a fever, these teas are a pleasant way to do so.

A fever over 102°F in an adult, or over 103°F in a child, that lasts for more than a day or so could indicate a serious illness that needs a doctor's attention.

❖ Flatulence

See Gas.

❖ Gallstones

Your gallbladder is a small, pear-shaped organ, about 3 to 6 inches long, that lies underneath the liver in the upper right side of the abdomen. The gallbladder serves as a reservoir for bile, a fluid made by the liver and used by the body to digest food. Small tubes called bile ducts connect the gallbladder to the liver and to the small intestine. Between meals, bile accumulates in the gallbladder. When you eat, the gallbladder contracts and empties the bile into the small intestine.

Excess cholesterol is removed from your blood by the liver and secreted into bile. When the bile contains too much cholesterol, small crystals form and the excess cholesterol falls to the bottom of the gallbladder. Eventually, the crystals form into gallstones. In most cases, the gallstones are harmless and asymptomatic. Sometimes, however, the stones cause irritation or even get lodged in the bile duct. In mild cases, gallstone symptoms include moderate pain in the upper part of the stomach and a bloated or full feeling. In more serious cases, the symptoms are severe, intermittent pain in the right upper abdomen (this pain is sometimes mistaken for a heart attack); chronic indigestion; and nausea. Gallstones are so common that about 10 percent of the population has them, although most of these people never know it. Even so, surgery to remove the gallbladder is now one of the most common operations.

Risk factors for developing gallstones include being obese (which increases your risk three to seven times), getting older, being a woman, being pregnant, taking hormonal birth control pills, taking estrogen for menopause, having a family history of gallstones, being of Native American ancestry, and having recently lost a lot of weight.

Herbalists refer to herbs that stimulate the production of bile or empty the gallbladder as cholagogues. Some of these herbs are safe and effective for relieving mild gallstone symptoms, although they should not be used for severe attacks or if symptoms persist. However, there is no real evidence that any herb can dissolve gallstones or keep them from forming.

Strong peppermint tea taken three or four times a day is a traditional remedy that can help. An alcoholic extract of peppermint (you can get this at a well-stocked pharmacy) can be used instead of tea; take 20 drops in 3 ounces of water up to four times a day. Gentian tea, made by steeping 1/2 teaspoon of ground root in 1/2 cup of boiling water for five minutes, can also relieve symptoms. Take it no more than four times a day.

Herbal mixtures, made into a strong tea and taken half an hour before meals, are sometimes recommended to help prevent gallbladder attacks. You could try combining equal parts peppermint leaves, chamomile flowers, and gentian root; some herbalists suggest adding fennel seeds.

Dandelion root, a traditional European gallstone remedy, is ineffective. Other herbs, such as yellow dock, yarrow, fennel, buckthorn, white oak bark, and rhubarb, have been recommended by herbalists, but there is little or no evidence that they are effective.

In India, turmeric, a yellow powder that is an essential ingredient in curry powder, has long been recommended as a cholagogue. Use an extract or tincture or take the herb in capsules to treat occasional indigestion accompanied by a bloated feeling, but do not use it if you have, or suspect, gallstones or a blocked bile duct. In fact, if you have gallstones, you should avoid curry powder.

There's not much evidence that diet has anything to do with causing gallstones (except, of course, that eating too much makes you obese) or that changing your diet to avoid fatty foods will cure the problem or prevent it. Some evidence shows that a diet high in fresh vegetables, nuts, beans, and legumes can help reduce your chances of gallbladder trouble. In this case, it's probably not just the fiber that helps. Researchers think that something in the vegetable protein can block or even dissolve the gallstones.

❖ Gas

A certain amount of intestinal gas is a normal by-product of digestion. In fact, the average person passes gas about fourteen times a day, for a volume of about a quart. Large amounts of gas, however, may be embarrassing or uncomfortable. Fortunately, there are some effective herbal ways to relieve the discomfort.

Some foods do produce more gas when digested than others. Beans, of course, are famous for producing flatulence, but don't let that stop you. Beans and lentils are a healthy and delicious way to add low-calorie, low-fat protein, carbohydrates, and fiber to your diet. Soak the beans well, then drain and rinse them before cooking. Despite what some old cookbooks say, don't add baking soda to the beans. It won't do anything about the gas and it makes the beans hard. Instead, add garlic or ginger to the beans. Many people claim these spices reduce the gas problem.

Herbs that relieve stomach or intestinal gas are known as carminatives. Most effective carminatives contain volatile oils that relax the muscles of the stomach or intestine, which allows the gas to pass through more easily.

The best-known and most effective carminative herbs are peppermint, chamomile, anise, caraway, and fennel. If you're having gas, try a cup or two of strong peppermint tea. If you prefer, an alcoholic extract of peppermint (you can get this at a well-stocked pharmacy) can be used in place of tea; take 20 drops in 3 ounces of water up to four times a day. Strong chamomile tea is also effective, but be sure you are getting a good product. Purchase whole dried flower heads; avoid powdered or crushed chamomile. Chamomile oil, which has a blue color, often contains adulterants that reduce its effectiveness; the tea is better.

Teas made from caraway, anise, or fennel seeds, which all have a characteristic licorice flavor, are safe and effective for relieving gas. Make a tea by crushing 1 teaspoonful of the seeds and steeping it in 1 cup of boiling water for fifteen minutes. Strain before drinking. Adding 5 to 10 drops of this tea to a baby's bottle can help relieve colicky gas pains.

Another herbal tea mixture that is often effective for flatulence is a combination of 3 parts chamomile and fennel seeds with 1 part chopped fresh gingerroot. Steep in boiling water for fifteen minutes and strain before drinking.

❖ Gingivitis
See Gum Disease.

❖ Glaucoma

Glaucoma is among the leading causes of blindness in the United States, affecting nearly three million people, yet it is a disease that can easily be detected and controlled. If you have glaucoma, the normal fluid pressure inside your eyes gradually rises, leading to vision loss or even blindness. The people most at risk for glaucoma are African-Americans over age forty (African-Americans between the ages of forty-five and sixty-five are fifteen times more likely to become blind from glaucoma than white Americans); anyone over age sixty; and people with a family history of glaucoma. You're also at risk if you are very nearsighted or have diabetes.

When glaucoma is detected early during a routine eye examination, the prospects for controlling the disease and preventing vision loss are very good. If you fall into one of the high-risk groups, the National Eye Institute recommends that you have your eyes examined through dilated pupils every two years. Glaucoma usually has no obvious symptoms until it has already damaged your eyes. There is no cure for glaucoma, but most people respond well to medication.

No evidence proves that taking the herbs eyebright, goldenseal, or yellow dock internally will help glaucoma. Never, under any circumstances, use any sort of herbal eyewash or eyedrops, homemade or purchased. Putting anything that isn't sterile into your eyes is dangerous and could cause infection; in addition, eyewashes or drops will wash away the eyedrops your doctor prescribes.

It's possible that taking supplemental vitamin C (500 milligrams daily) may help reduce eye pressure in people with glaucoma. Some preliminary animal research suggests that fish oil (omega-3 fatty acids) may also reduce eye pressure. Some evidence shows that a concentrated extract of the anthocyanosides found in dried blueberries or bilberries may protect against glaucoma. You can't get the required concentration from eating dried blueberries, but research in this area is promising. If you are at risk for glaucoma or already have it, take your medicine and discuss taking extra vitamin C and fish oil supplements with your doctor.

❖ Gout

Gout, a form of arthritis, is caused by an excess of uric acid in the blood. Crystals of the acid get deposited in the joints, particularly the big toe, causing the joint to swell up and be extremely painful. Gout is almost exclusively a disease of men: over 90 percent of people with gout are male.

The pain of gout attacks can be relieved with drugs, including nonsteroidal anti-inflammatories such as ibuprofen. The best treatment, however, is prevention through diet. Eliminate alcohol, which prevents your body from excreting uric acid, and lose weight—more than half of all gout sufferers are overweight. Most importantly, avoid eating foods that contain purine, since uric acid is produced when these foods are digested. Meats, particularly organ meats, and seafood are very high in purine. Some foods and herbs often recommended by herbalists are also moderately high in purine. These include bran, celery, hawthorn berries, mushrooms, oatmeal, rhubarb, spinach, and wheat germ. These foods should be eaten only in moderation; if gout symptoms still occur, avoid them.

Fluids help dilute the uric acid in the blood, so gout patients should drink at least two quarts a day. Some people with gout find that eating cherries, blueberries, or strawberries (or drinking juice made from these fruits) every day helps prevent attacks. During a gout attack, a traditional herbal remedy is strong tea made from crushed celery seeds. Use 1 teaspoonful of seeds to 1 cup boiling water; let steep for fifteen minutes, then strain and drink. Repeat up to three times a day until the attack subsides.

Numerous other herbs, some with mild diuretic effects, have traditionally been recommended by herbalists for gout. Teas made from horsetail, vervain, burdock root, dandelion root, pennyroyal, red clover flowers, and yucca may be helpful, if only because drinking a lot of fluids is helpful.

❖ Gum Disease

The two most common gum (periodontal) diseases are gingivitis and periodontitis (sometimes called pyorrhea). Gingivitis is an infection of the gums that causes them to become red and inflamed; they may bleed when you brush your teeth.

Gingivitis is caused by the buildup of plaque—a sticky mass of harmful germs—on your teeth. You can usually get rid of gingivitis by improving your dental hygiene. To prevent plaque buildup, brush your teeth twice a day, floss daily, and have your teeth cleaned professionally at least once a year.

If it is not treated, gingivitis can progress until it becomes a more destructive type of gum disease called periodontitis. This is an infection of the tissues that help anchor your teeth into your jaw. Signs of periodontitis include painful, bleeding gums, abcesses, and bad breath. The infection can lead to loss of the bone that holds the tooth in its socket, which in turn could lead to tooth loss. Since periodontitis affects more than just the gums, better dental hygiene won't solve the problem. Treatment from a dentist or a periodontist (a dentist who specializes in treating gum diseases), such as scaling to remove plaque and planing to smooth the tooth root, are effective. Your dentist may also recommend a special mouthwash containing chlorhexidine. If deep pockets of infection have developed around your teeth, gum surgery may be necessary.

Some herbs can help prevent the buildup of dental plaque if they are used in combination with good dental hygiene. Bloodroot contains antibacterial compounds that help keep bacteria from sticking to your teeth. Extracts of bloodroot are often added to natural toothpastes and mouthwashes. You can also buy bloodroot extract at a health food store. Dilute it 10 to 1 in water for a homemade antiplaque mouthwash. Chewing on fresh basil leaves is an old European treatment for plaque that is mildly effective. Myrrh, a fragrant resin known since ancient times, is sometimes used as an antiseptic and flavoring ingredient in commercial mouthwashes. You can make your own version by diluting myrrh tincture 10 to 1 in water. Strong teas of vervain, goldenseal, calendula, or horsetail may help relieve gingivitis symptoms when they are used as mouthwashes; betony (also called wood betony) is also effective. In India, people chew on neem twigs to clean their teeth and freshen their breath; fresh curry leaves are used for the same purpose.

See also Mouth Sores; Tooth Care.

❖ Hangover

Generations of drinkers have passed along numerous herbal folk cures, but the sad fact is that there is nothing that will cure a hangover once you've had too much to drink. The only question is what you can do to relieve the headache and nausea that are inevitable symptoms.

To reduce the severity of a hangover, simply drink less or drink more slowly. Avoid whiskey and other dark liquors and stick to clear alcohol such as vodka. Also avoid carbonated mixers, beer, sparkling wine, and red wine.

Because alcohol has a dehydrating effect, try drinking a large glass of water or fruit juice before going to bed. Repeat the treatment in the morning. The liquid replenishes the lost fluids; the fructose in fruit juice may also help you metabolize the alcohol in your system. To help relieve morning-after symptoms, some herbalists recommend skullcap or valerian root tea; others say two evening primrose oil or borage seed oil capsules will help. So does a cup or two of hot coffee. Strong hot peppermint or chamomile tea can help relieve nausea and indigestion. In traditional Chinese herbal medicine, ginseng tea is used as a hangover remedy. An old Italian folk remedy suggests strong hot chicken broth served with lots of garlic and dandelion leaves. Some natural medicine practitioners now recommend taking two or three evening primrose oil capsules the next morning.

❖ Hay Fever

Hay fever, also known as allergic rhinitis, is an allergic reaction to pollen and other airborne substances such as house dust and mold. According to the National Institute of Allergy and Infectious Disease, hay fever affects some thirty-five million Americans, causing them to sneeze, sniffle, and have itchy, runny eyes.

Pollen from ragweed is one of the most common causes of hay fever, but pollen from many other plants can also be culprits, especially weeds such as sagebrush and lamb's quarters; such trees as oak, ash, hickory, elm, pecan, box elder, and mountain cedar; and such grasses as timothy, Bermuda, and Kentucky bluegrass. Despite its name, hay fever is rarely caused by hay; rose fever, an old-fashioned name for hay fever, is also misleading, because pollen from colorful or scented flowers rarely causes allergic reactions.

There is no cure for airborne allergies. Avoiding pollen, house dust, and mold will help reduce hay fever symptoms, but these substances are often so prevalent that exposure is inevitable. Staying in an air-conditioned space can help, as can some kinds of air filters. Smoking, or being in a smoky environment, and drinking alcohol can seriously aggravate your hay fever—avoid them.

If you have severe hay fever, some herbal remedies could trigger an allergic response. Try to avoid herbs made from flowers, such as chamomile, red clover, chickweed, golden-rod, and lamb's quarters. Also avoid bee pollen and royal jelly. Eyebright is often recommended as a treatment for hay fever, but it is unlikely to do much good; do not use it or any other herbal preparation as an eyewash for itchy or runny eyes. Ephedra, also called ma huang in traditional Chinese medicine, can be effective for hay fever symptoms, especially wheeziness or coughing. (Mormon tea, an herb related to ephedra, is ineffective for hay fever, so be sure you are getting the right herb.) If you have a dry cough or tickle in your throat from hay fever, try a tea made from Iceland moss. Some hay fever sufferers claim that eating a cup or two a day of live-culture yogurt helps ward off their symptoms. Others say that eating lots of onions helps; the antioxidant substance quercetin in the onions may help block the allergic response.

If herbs don't help, ask your doctor or pharmacist about antihistamines to help control the symptoms. Some of the newer antihistamines are very effective and do not cause drowsiness, dry mouth, or other unwanted side effects. Allergy shots (immunotherapy) can often help reduce the severity of allergic reactions.

See also Asthma.

❖ Headaches

According to the National Headache Foundation, each year forty-five million Americans get headaches that are bad enough to seek the help of a doctor. Several different types of headaches may be brought on by a variety of different causes, but the most common type by far—about 90 percent of all headaches—is the tension headache, characterized by dull pain and a feeling of tightness around the scalp and neck. Most tension headaches are caused by stress, fatigue, or depression.

Almost any sort of mild herbal tea, sweetened with a spoonful of honey if you wish, can help relieve a tension headache. This is probably because taking the time to make the tea and sip it in a quiet place provides a break from the stress, while the tea itself has an overall soothing effect. Favorite herbs for tension headaches include lavender, peppermint, chamomile, lemon balm, rose hips, and ginger. Another use for these herbal teas is to let them cool and then make a cold compress. Lie down in a quiet, dark place and place the compress on your forehead; leave it there for ten minutes and repeat if necessary. Instead of a compress, try rubbing a few drops of peppermint or lavender oil into your temples.

Rosemary tea is a traditional remedy in Europe that is said to relieve headaches and provide an energy boost at the same time. Willow bark is said to be effective because it contains salicylates, which are similar to aspirin. Since willow bark tea is bitter and slow to act, however, try taking the powdered form in capsules. Ginseng tea is the headache remedy typically suggested in traditional Chinese herbal medicine. Valerian tea has a calming effect that is very helpful for tension headaches, but it may also make you sleepy. If you have a tension headache but want to stay alert, try relaxing for ten minutes over a hot cup of coffee or tea. A favorite South American remedy, a relaxing cup of maté, also contains caffeine.

Some headaches are brought on by hunger, not tension. Hunger headaches usually start just before mealtime. They're caused by a combination of muscle tension and low blood sugar, and are far more likely to occur when you're dieting or skipping meals. Here the solution is obvious: good, nutritious meals eaten on a regular basis. The hunger headaches will go away, and you'll feel better in general.

Caffeine withdrawal headaches are very common. Most people who drink caffeinated beverages daily and then break the routine by skipping a day will get a mild headache. The headache generally goes away when you get some caffeine. If you're trying to cut back on caffeine, taper off gradually to avoid withdrawal headaches.

Some foods and food additives cause headaches in sensitive people. Monosodium glutamate (MSG), a very common food additive, is a well-known headache trigger. Read all food labels carefully, since MSG is commonly used in a wide variety of preapred foods. It's also found in seasoned salts, meat tenderizers, and soy sauce. The food additives sodium nitrite and sodium nitrate can also cause headaches. These substances are very often added to prepared meats such as hot dogs, bacon, salami, and ham. The artificial sweetener aspartame (NutraSweet) can cause headaches in some sensitive people.

Cluster headaches, a relatively rare but very painful ailment, begin suddenly and unexpectedly; the pain is around or behind one eye. They're so named because attacks occur in clusters or groups for days, weeks, or even months at a time and then may disappear completely for a year or more. See your doctor at once if you have cluster headaches.

See also Migraine.

❖ Hearing Problems

See Tinnitus.

❖ Heart Attack

Heart attack is the leading cause of death in the United States. Annually about 1.5 million Americans have one; of those, nearly 490,000 will die. A heart attack (also known as a myocardial infarction or coronary) occurs when one of the coronary arteries, which supply blood to the heart, becomes greatly narrowed or blocked. As a result, part of the heart muscle doesn't get the oxygen it needs and begins to die.

High blood pressure, high blood cholesterol, cigarette smoking, and lack of physical activity are the major risk factors for heart attacks; other risk facors include obesity and diabetes. Having a family history of heart disease, being male, being African-American, and just getting older are additional risk factors.

Can the omega-3 fatty acids found in fish oil, especially from deep sea fish such as mackerel, salmon, anchovies, herring, tuna, and sardines, help prevent a heart attack? Since the mid-1980s, doctors have suggested that people at risk for heart attacks eat 5 ounces of fish twice a week to help their blood flow better, open arteries, prevent clotting, lower blood pressure, and raise HDL (good) cholesterol levels. In addition, some people took supplemental fish oil capsules. In 1995, however, the results of a large-scale study by the Harvard School of Public Health showed that eating more fish did not, in fact, lower the risk of heart attack for healthy men between the ages of forty and seventy-five.

Today, almost all doctors recommend that heart patients eat a variety of foods that are high in fiber and low in fat, which means lots of fresh fruits and vegetables. Add an onion, plenty of garlic, and a handful of unsalted nuts daily to help prevent blood clots and keep your arteries open. No more than 30 percent of your daily calories should come from fat—and avoid animal fat. Instead, substitute monounsaturated fats such as olive oil or canola oil. Studies show that monounsaturated fats can actually help protect your arteries against damage.

Traditionally, herbal remedies based on hawthorn flowers and berries have been recommended in Europe for treating heart disease. Some hawthorn formulations are commercially available in Europe, but the benefits of hawthorn remain unproven. Various other herbs are sometimes recommended as heart tonics. These include lobelia, lily of the valley, motherwort, and ginseng. If you are at risk for a heart attack or have already had one, do not attempt to treat yourself with hawthorn or other herbs.

Heart Attack Warning Signs

Since nearly one-third of all heart attacks are fatal, someone having a heart attack needs immediate medical help. Look for these warning signs:

- An uncomfortable feeling of pressure, fullness, squeezing, or pain in the center of the chest that lasts for more than a few minutes
- Pain that spreads or radiates to the shoulders, neck, or arm (especially down the left arm)
- Chest discomfort along with feeling lightheaded, shortness of breath, fainting, sweating, or nausea

See also Angina; Atherosclerosis.

❖ Heartburn

A painful burning feeling in your upper stomach, along with a sour or bitter taste in your throat or mouth, is called heartburn or sour stomach. Heartburn has nothing to do with your heart—it's your esophagus, a 10-inch tube that leads from your mouth to your stomach, that's causing the trouble.

When you eat, food passes down the esophagus and into your stomach through a ringlike opening called the lower esophageal sphincter. The ring opens to allow the food in, and then closes again to keep your acid digestive juices in your stomach. Sometimes, however, the ring doesn't close completely or doesn't stay closed. Food and stomach acid then back up (reflux) into the esophagus, causing the burning sensation of heartburn.

Occasional heartburn is very common. Eating too much or eating too quickly are the most likely causes, but often how you eat isn't the problem; it's what you eat. Certain foods such as chocolate, onions, fatty or fried foods, and alcohol relax the sphincter muscles and make reflux more likely. Other foods such as juices, coffee, carbonated drinks such as soda pop and beer, and milk, can increase the amount of acid your stomach produces, creating the same effect. Acidic foods such as tomato juice, tomatoes, citrus juice, coffee, and some spicy foods may irritate the esophagus and make the existing problem worse. Heartburn can sometimes be a side effect of medications. If you think your medicine is causing heartburn, talk to your doctor or pharmacist.

Fortunately, some simple remedies for heartburn are very effective. The simplest of all is to just drink a glass of cold water. This can wash the acid back into your stomach and relieve the pain. Some claim that the juice of a raw potato, mixed half and half with water, does wonders. Others say that drinking 1 tablespoon of apple cider vinegar mixed into 8 ounces of water during meals keeps them from getting heartburn. A cup of strong, hot peppermint tea is often very effective. Strong chamomile tea is also effective, but be sure you are getting a good product. Purchase whole dried flower heads; avoid powdered or crushed chamomile.

Teas made from caraway, anise, or fennel seeds are also safe and effective for relieving heartburn. They all have a characteristic licorice flavor. Make them into teas by crushing 1 teaspoonful of the seeds and steeping it in 1 cup of boiling water for fifteen minutes. Strain before drinking. Tea made from lemon balm helps some people as well.

If you get heartburn often, try making a strong tea from equal parts peppermint leaves, chamomile flowers, and gentian root, along with a pinch of crushed fennel seeds. Drink a cup after eating to help prevent heartburn symptoms.

There are some other practical steps you can take to reduce how often you get heartburn. Lose weight if you are too heavy. If you smoke, stop. Avoid tight-fitting clothing that puts pressure on your abdomen. Don't lie down right after eating. Instead, wait two or three hours. Many people find that elevating the head of the bed by about six inches helps relieve reflux problems.

Heartburn may be a symptom of a more serious problem such as gallstones or ulcers. If your heartburn is very severe, or if you have it more frequently than three times a week over a period of two weeks, call your doctor. Other danger signs include difficulty or pain when swallowing, vomiting blood, bloody or black stools, shortness of breath, dizziness or lightheadedness, pain going into your neck and shoulder, or breaking out into a sweat when you have the pain.

See also Ulcers.

❖ Hemorrhoids

Hemorrhoids are an extremely common ailment causing pain, itching, and discomfort to some twenty-five million Americans. Hemorrhoids occur when the veins in the lower rectum, at the junction with the anal canal, become swollen and bulge out beneath the thin layer of tissue that covers them. *Internal hemorrhoids* occur in the upper portion of the anal canal and may cause pain, burning, itching, or aching in the area. These hemorrhoids may also bleed, leaving bright red blood on the stool or on the toilet paper after a movement. *External hemorrhoids* occur under the surface of the skin at the anal opening. They tend to disappear after a few days, but then come back. External hemorrhoids produce pain, swelling, burning, and itching of the overlying skin.

Anything that puts stress and pressure on the network of delicate hemorrhoidal veins can cause this condition. A low-fiber, high-fat diet is the major culprit, because it leads to constipation or straining during bowel movements. Lack of exercise, sitting or standing for long periods, being overweight, or doing a lot of lifting are other contributing factors. Pregnant women often develop hemorrhoids because of the weight and pressure of the growing baby. These hemorrhoids usually go away after the baby is born.

In most cases, you can easily treat your hemorrhoid symptoms yourself. Sitz baths or warm compresses can be very helpful. Pain and itching can be relieved by applying plain petroleum jelly, witch hazel, or nonprescription creams to the area. Herbal creams made from calendula are often helpful. An oil made from St. John's wort is used in Europe as an external treatment and is quite effective. This reddish oil can be purchased in well-stocked health food stores. Another European herbal treatment that is becoming popular in the United States is bucher's broom, in ointment or suppository form. This herb contains compounds that help constrict swollen blood vessels and may also have anti-inflammatory properties.

The best treatment for hemorrhoids, however, is to avoid constipation and straining by eating a high-fiber diet. The fiber makes your stool softer and bulkier so that it passes much more easily. If you wish, try using bulk-forming laxatives. Psyllium seed husks, also called plantago seed, is the ingredient found in over-the-counter bulk-forming laxatives such as Metamucil.

Some people find that particular foods, such as coffee or nuts, aggravate their hemorrhoids; very spicy foods or foods with a lot of ginger can also cause problems. Needless to say, if you notice that something you eat or drink makes your hemorrhoids worse, avoid it. Drinking plenty of liquids—six to eight glasses a day—and getting regular exercise also promote regularity.

If your hemorrhoids are very painful or bleeding a lot, call your doctor.

❖ Hepatitis

Hepatitis means simply inflammation of the liver. In most cases, hepatitis is caused by a virus; in some cases, it is caused by toxins such as drugs or alcohol. The symptoms can vary a lot from person to person. They can be mild enough not to be noticed, or they can be easily confused with an intestinal flu. The early signs are quite similar to flu: fatigue, joint and muscle pain, and loss of appetite. Later on, you may be nauseous, vomit, have diarrhea, and run a low-grade fever. Your liver (the upper right side of your abdomen) may feel tender, and you may develop jaundice (yellow skin).

Five different kinds of viral hepatitis have been identified. In the United States, the most common form (more than half of all cases) is hepatitis A (sometimes called infectious hepatitis). The virus is excreted through the feces, so it is usually spread by poor hygiene. Epidemics of hepatitis A can be spread when food, water, or shellfish beds are contaminated. Hepatitis B (also called serum hepatitis) infects about 300,000 people in the United States every year. The virus is found in all the body fluids of the infected person. Hepatitis B is usually spread by intimate contact with an infected person, although it can also spread through contaminated instruments used for tattooing, body piercing, drug injection, and the like. The other forms of hepatitis—C, D, and E—are less common. Hepatitis C (also called non-A, non-B hepatitis) affects some 150,000 Americans every year. It is primarily spread through blood transfusions. Hepatitis D is a liver infection found only in conjunction with hepatitis B. Hepatitis E (sometimes called epidemic or waterborne hepatitis), is spread by contaminated water. So far, it is not a common illness in America, but epidemics have occurred in Mexico.

Hepatitis A and B usually clear up by themselves in about a month to six weeks, although it may take three or four months before you feel completely yourself again. The best treatment is rest and a good diet. Most doctors recommend a diet that is low in fat, dairy products, and sugar, high in complex carbohydrates and fresh fruits and vegetables, and has absolutely no alcohol. Don't take acetaminophen (Tylenol) or ibuprofen (Advil). These drugs could cause liver damage. If you take other prescription or nonprescription drugs, discuss them with your doctor.

Eating well can be a big problem for hepatitis patients due to nausea and loss of appetite. Try eating frequent small meals instead of three large ones. Drink plenty of liquids. In addition, take a daily multivitamin and get some extra vitamin A and all the B vitamins to help your liver recover faster. Don't overdo it, however. Too much vitamin A is toxic to your liver.

Silymarin, an antioxidant flavonoid found in milk thistle, may have a beneficial effect on the liver by stimulating the production of new liver cells; this herb is under active scientific investigation. Herbalists recommend that silymarin be taken in the form of milk thistle capsules, found in health food stores, as milk thistle tea does not have a high enough concentration of active ingredients. Schisandra, a remedy for liver problems in traditional Chinese herbal medicine, is said to have a protective effect on the liver. Researchers are studying the active ingredients in schisandra fruit, but the results so far are inconclusive. Dandelion leaves and roots are a traditional herbal remedy for hepatitis, but they are ineffective. Other herbal remedies that have been suggested over the years include artichoke leaf tea, burdock root, red clover flowers, and licorice. Again, none are effective. Spirulina, or green alga, is said to help hepatitis, but there is no evidence that supports this. The amino acid arginine, which is found naturally in many foods, including chocolate, nuts, seeds, whole grains, corn, and beer, is sometimes said to be a liver cleanser. However, there is no proof that taking supplemental arginine will help you get over hepatitis faster.

Hepatitis A and B usually go away without any long-term effects; the other types are more likely to have serious complications, among them, lifelong liver disease. Even mild hepatitis, however, can lead to serious problems. If you think you have hepatitis, see your doctor at once.

❖ Herpes

Herpes simplex type 1 (HSV-1), the virus that causes cold sores, is closely related to herpes simplex type 2 (HSV-2), the virus that causes genital herpes. Both forms of herpes simplex cause painful blisters and sores. Genital herpes has become a very common sexually transmitted disease. About 16 percent of all Americans between the ages of fifteen and seventy-four have HSV-2—that's about thirty million people, or one in every six.

The unmistakable symptoms of genital herpes usually develop within two days to three weeks. At first, there is usually redness and inflammation in the genital area; next, one or more blisters or bumps appear. The blisters quickly break and become painful open sores. The area is usually very painful and may itch, burn, or tingle. Often, flulike symptoms—swollen glands, headache, muscle aches, or fever—accompany the outbreak. During this time, even before the blisters appear, and whenever herpes sores are present, avoid intercourse. Even a latex condom may not protect your partner. To protect your partner at all other times, always use a condom.

A first attack of genital herpes can last for several weeks. Eventually, the area heals up and the symptoms subside, but the herpes virus never really goes away. Some people have only occasional, mild flare-ups, but many people have recurrences more frequently, often four or more times a year. Fortunately, recurrences are usually far less severe than the initial attack, and they generally get less severe with time.

To treat the painful sores, avoid any sort of cream, ointment, or petroleum jelly, because these can trap bacteria and cause infection. Antibiotic creams will have no effect on the virus anyway, while cortisone creams could actually encourage viral growth. To help the sores heal, keep the area clean with plain soap and water; try to expose it to the air as much as possible. Applying fresh aloe vera gel to the sores may provide some temporary relief; some people use diluted tea tree oil. Warm compresses applied to the sores can be very helpful for relieving the pain of an outbreak. You can soak the compress in plain warm water or in tea made from yellow dock, goldenseal, white oak bark, or chamomile. Some herpes sufferers say that taking garlic capsules helps shorten their outbreaks; others say that goldenseal, taken in capsules or as a strong tea, is helpful.

Many people with genital herpes say that stress, illness, fatigue, being out in the sun, menstruation, or eating certain foods triggers their outbreaks. Some people claim that coffee, alcohol, sugary foods, colas, or yeast trigger recurrences. There's no real evidence one way or the other, but if you notice a correlation, by all means avoid the triggering substance.

Many people have tried using dietary supplements of the amino acid lysine to control genital herpes attacks. Lysine is found in milk, yogurt, eggs, cheese, and meat. Scientific studies have produced mixed results, but some people say that lysine supplements help them. Another amino acid, arginine, has been implicated in outbreaks in some people. Foods rich in arginine include chocolate, nuts, seeds, whole grains, corn, and beer. Again, the scientific evidence for this is slim, but avoiding arginine seems to work for some people. Some evidence has shown that eating a diet rich in vitamin A and iron can help reduce recurrences.

Most physicians feel that a nutritious, well-balanced diet is the best defense against herpes recurrences. Avoid alcohol, since drinking can reduce your nutritional status and depress your immune system. A daily multivitamin supplement is probably a good idea, but expensive megadose vitamin therapy is generally worthless and can even be harmful.

For more information about genital herpes, contact the National Herpes Hotline at 919/361-8488 or the Herpes Resource Center at 800/230-6039.

❖ Hiatus Hernia

Your esophagus (the tube that leads from your mouth to your stomach) passes through an opening, a hiatus, in your diaphragm. (Your diaphragm is a dome-shaped sheet of muscle separating your abdomen from your chest that moves up and down as you breathe.) If you have a hiatus hernia, the muscles around the hiatus have weakened and allowed the abdominal part of your esophagus, and sometimes the upper part of your stomach, to protrude up into your chest cavity.

Hiatus hernia is quite common, particularly among overweight, older people. It's often symptomless, but some people get painful acid reflux—better known as heartburn—if stomach acid is pushed up into the esophagus.

Several self-help steps can relieve hiatus hernia problems. If you are overweight, lose weight. Because lying down flat lets stomach acid flow more easily up into your esophagus, elevate the head of your bed by 6 inches or so (raise the bed itself—don't use pillows). Avoid tight clothing, stooping, and lying down immediately after eating. Many people find that eating several small meals a day instead of two of three large ones helps relieve their symptoms. Alcohol and tobacco usually worsen hiatus hernia symptoms and should be avoided.

For more information on how to relieve the symptoms of acid reflux, see the section on Heartburn.

❖ High Blood Pressure

Every time your heart beats (about sixty to seventy times a minute when you are resting), it pumps blood out to the arteries, which carry the blood away from your heart to the rest of your body. Blood pressure is the force of that blood as it pushes against the walls of the arteries. Your blood pressure is highest when the heart contracts and pushes blood out—the systolic pressure. When the heart is at rest between beats, your blood pressure falls—the diastolic pressure. When your blood pressure is taken, the result is always given as two numbers: the systolic and diastolic pressure. The measurement is written one above or before the other, with the systolic number on top or first.

Normal blood pressure ranges anywhere from below 130 up to 140 systolic and from below 85 up to 90 diastolic. If your blood pressure is less than 140/90, then, it is considered normal. High blood pressure, or hypertension, is anything above 140/90 and is classified by stages; it gets more serious as the numbers get higher.

For most people, hypertension has no single known cause. This type of high blood pressure is called essential hypertension. Although it can't be cured, in most cases it can be controlled. Uncontrolled high blood pressure can lead to arteriosclerosis (hardening of the arteries), heart attack, enlarged heart, kidney damage, or stroke. High blood pressure itself generally has no symptoms or warning signs. The only way to know if you have it is to have your blood pressure checked regularly. If it is high, you can take steps to lower it.

If your blood pressure is normal, you can learn how to keep it that way.

Anyone can develop high blood pressure. There are some important steps you can take, however, to help prevent the problem or control the problem:

- Maintain a healthy weight. Lose weight if you are too heavy.
- Be more physically active.
- Choose foods that are lower in salt and sodium.
- Choose foods that are lower in saturated fats.
- Drink alcoholic beverages in moderation—no more than two drinks a day.
- If you smoke, stop.

Salt and sodium strongly affect the blood pressure of some people and not of others, although it's not clear why. If you have high blood pressure, it's best to be on the safe side. Try to limit your salt intake to 2,400 milligrams (about a teaspoon) a day. Try substituting other seasonings, such as garlic, onion, lemon juice, and other flavorful herbs and spices, for the salt. Remember that salt is widely used in many prepared and processed foods and is also a major ingredient in condiments such as steak sauce.

Many researchers feel that a diet high in omega-3 fatty acids can help prevent or lower high blood pressure. Omega-3 fatty acids, also called fish oils, are found in deep ocean fatty fish such as salmon, mackeral, anchovies, sardines, herring, and tuna. Many doctors recommend that patients with high blood pressure eat a small portion of fatty fish two or three times a week or take supplemental fish oil capsules. It might also be a good idea to substitute olive oil for other oils in your diet. This monounsaturated fat seems to help lower blood pressure.

If you already have high blood pressure, your doctor may suggest that you avoid caffeine. If you don't have high blood pressure, however, there is no evidence that caffeine will cause it.

Some evidence suggests that certain minerals can affect high blood pressure. Eating foods rich in potassium appears to protect some people. Population studies have shown that populations with low calcium intakes have high rates of high blood pressure. While it is unclear if taking calcium supplements will prevent high blood pressure, eating a diet rich in calcium-containing foods will at least ensure that you get enough. Magnesium is another mineral that affects your blood pressure. Too little magnesium can make your blood pressure go up. Again, doctors caution against taking supplemental magnesium; instead, get your recommended dietary allowance of 300 to 350 milligrams a day by eating dark green leafy vegetables, nuts, seeds, and whole grains. They are good sources of potassium, magnesium, and calcium. Alfalfa sprouts are a very good choice for all minerals, while dandelion leaves and watercress contain calcium and magnesium.

If you have mild high blood pressure, eating a couple of celery stalks or some fresh parsley leaves every day can be helpful. Garlic and onions contain adenosine, which relaxes the blood vessels and makes them open up, lowering blood pressure. The fiber in all fruits and vegetables seems to have an overall beneficial effect on your blood pressure as well. However, these foods are not substitutes for taking your prescribed blood pressure medication.

Doctors often prescribe diuretic drugs for patients with high blood pressure. These drugs keep you from retaining fluids by making you excrete more urine, which in turn helps lower your blood pressure. Many traditional herbal remedies for high blood pressure, such as dandelion root, black cohosh, goldenrod, and bearberry (uva ursi), also have a diuretic effect. Increased urination, however, may also deplete your body of essential minerals, particularly potassium and sodium. Modern diuretic drugs prevent mineral depletion, but herbal medicines do not. If you take an herbal diuretic instead of, or in addition to, a diuretic your doctor prescribes, you could seriously disturb your body's mineral balance, with possibly fatal consequences. If you have high blood pressure, talk to your doctor before you try any herbal treatment.

In traditional Chinese herbal medicine, ginseng is suggested for lowering high blood pressure. This may be beneficial for very mild hypertension, but you should still take any medication your doctor prescribes. A traditional European herbal treatment for high blood pressure is mistletoe leaves. However, this is not effective and the leaves contain toxic compounds that could be dangerous. Don't use them.

Warning: Do not use any herbal remedies containing licorice if you have high blood pressure. This could raise your blood pressure higher. Also avoid herbal remedies containing goldenseal, yohimbe, or ephedra (also called ma huang). These herbs can also raise your blood pressure.

See also Diabetes; Dialysis.

❖ High Cholesterol

Cholesterol, a waxy, fatty substance found in all parts of your body, is essential for making your cell membranes, some hormones, and vitamin D. The cholesterol in your body comes from two sources: your body and your food. Blood cholesterol is made by your liver; in fact, your liver makes all the cholesterol you need. Dietary cholesterol comes from animal foods such as meat, poultry, eggs, fish, and milk and dairy products. (Plant foods have no cholesterol.) Eating too many foods high in cholesterol can make your blood cholesterol level go up, and the higher it goes, the greater your chance of coronary heart disease. Excess cholesterol in your blood builds up on the walls of the arteries that carry blood to your heart. This buildup of fatty plaque, called atherosclerosis, narrows or even sometimes blocks the arteries that bring oxygen to the heart muscle. The eventual result is angina or a heart attack. Lowering your blood cholesterol level can slow the buildup of plaque; in some cases, it can even help reduce the buildup that is already there.

LDL vs. HDL

Just like oil and water, cholesterol and blood don't mix. So that cholesterol can travel throughout your body in the blood, it is coated with a layer of protein, forming a lipoprotein. There are several different kinds of lipoproteins, but the two most important are low-density lipoprotein (LDL) and high-density lipoprotein (HDL). Most of the cholesterol in your blood is carried as LDL cholesterol; only about a third to a quarter is carried as HDL cholesterol. Too much LDL cholesterol in the blood can lead to cholesterol buildup in the arteries. That's why LDL cholesterol is often called bad cholesterol. HDL cholesterol actually helps to remove cholesterol from the blood and to prevent the fatty buildup. That's why it is often called good cholesterol. Optimally, the goal is to lower your LDL (bad) level and raise your HDL (good) level.

A number of uncontrollable factors, such as age, sex, and heredity, influence your blood cholesterol level. Blood cholesterol levels in both men and women begin to rise around age twenty. Premenopausal women generally have lower cholesterol levels than men of the same age. After menopause, however, a woman's LDL level tends to go up. Having close relatives with high levels of LDL cholesterol or a history of heart disease increases the chances that your body is more likely to make a lot of LDL cholesterol and deposit it in your arteries.

You can't do much about your age, sex, or heredity, but you can do something about your diet, weight, and activity level. What you eat has a big effect on your cholesterol level. If you eat a lot of saturated fats or dietary cholesterol, you can elevate your cholesterol levels. Being overweight can also raise your level of LDL (bad) cholesterol and lower your HDL (good) level. On the other hand, increasing your level of physical activity can lower your LDL cholesterol level and raise your HDL level.

To measure your blood cholesterol levels, your doctor will take a fasting blood sample and send it to a laboratory. The levels are measured in milligrams per deciliter, abbreviated as mg/dL. The chart below explains the results.

Any total blood cholesterol level of 200 mg/dL or more increases your risk of heart disease. A level of 240 mg/dL or greater is considered high cholesterol and more than doubles your risk of heart disease as compared with someone who has a desirable cholesterol level. Unlike total cholesterol, where a lower number is better, the higher your HDL (good) cholesterol number, the better.

Blood Cholesterol Levels

Total Blood Cholesterol/HDL Cholesterol

Level	Category
Less than 35 mg/dL	Low
36–200 mg/dL	Desirable
200–239 mg/dL	Borderline high
240 mg/dL	High

LDL Cholesterol

Level	Category
Less than 130 mg/dL	Desirable
130–159 mg/dL	Borderline high risk
160 mg/dL and above	High risk

Lowering Your Cholesterol

If your cholesterol levels are too high, your doctor will recommend that you eat foods low in saturated fat and dietary cholesterol, get more exercise, and lose weight if necessary. He or she may also recommend medication in some cases, but diet and exercise are the most important steps you can take. Lowering your high cholesterol even a little can have a positive effect. A healthy forty-year-old man with borderline high cholesterol (200 to 240 mg/dL) who lowers his cholesterol by just ten percent can cut his risk of a heart attack by 50 percent. In other words, by making some simple changes in his diet, he can cut his chances of having a heart attack in half.

On average, Americans get 12 percent of their calories from saturated fat and 34 percent of their calories from total fat. The average daily intake of dietary cholesterol ranges from 220 to 260 milligrams for women and about 360 milligrams for men. These intakes are too high for most people. The National Cholesterol Education Program recommends that you get less than 10 percent of your calories from saturated fat, 30 percent or less of your calories from total fat, and eat less than 30 milligrams a day of dietary cholesterol. If you follow these guidelines, also known as the Step I diet, your blood cholesterol levels will probably fall over the course of several months. If the Step I diet isn't working, or if your cholesterol levels are very high, you might want to follow an even lower-fat diet, also known as the Step II diet. In this diet, less than 7 percent of your daily calories comes from saturated fat; 30 percent or less of your daily calories comes from total fat, and you eat less than 200 milligrams of dietary cholesterol in a day.

Changing your diet can help lower your blood cholesterol if it is too high, but it probably won't do much if your cholesterol level is normal or only slightly elevated. To lower your blood cholesterol, choose foods that are low in saturated fats, low in total fat, and low in dietary cholesterol. In general, lowering your intake of saturated fat is a lot more important than lowering your dietary cholesterol intake, but you should try to reduce both.

Adding fiber, particularly soluble fiber, to your diet can help you reduce your cholesterol level. In general, eating lots of fresh fruits and vegetables and cooked dried beans and peas has a beneficial effect. So does eating soybeans and other soy foods, such as bean curd (tofu) and soy milk, with the exception of soy sauce. Another excellent source of soluble fiber is oat bran, either by itself or as part of oatmeal. Just two ounces of oat bran a day (or one large bowl of oatmeal daily) can not only lower your LDL level, it can also raise your HDL level. The process takes a few months, and it may not work for everyone, but it's certainly worth trying if your cholesterol levels are high.

Onions and garlic contain substances that also seem to help reduce overall cholesterol and raise HDL levels. Raw onions and garlic seem to be the most effective. Some physicians now recommend half a raw onion or several raw garlic cloves (or garlic capsules) daily. Additional evidence suggests that people who drink Chinese green tea or oolong tea have lower cholesterol levels. If you have high cholesterol, try drinking a cup or two of Chinese tea each day instead of coffee or black tea.

Some herbalists claim that eating ginger or licorice can help lower cholesterol levels, but so far there isn't much evidence to support this. Another unsupported claim is that eating alfalfa (as tablets, liquid, or sprouts) before a meal will keep you from absorbing cholesterol.

Monounsaturated fats, such as olive oil, canola oil, and peanut oil, can help lower your blood cholesterol level. Olive oil contains antioxidant compounds that can help reduce oxidation of the LDL cholesterol in your blood. Similar compounds seem to be in the oils found in avocados and nuts such as walnuts and almonds. These foods aren't magic bullets, but the evidence suggests that substituting olive oil for other fats or eating a handful of walnuts instead of cookies as a snack could certainly help lower your cholesterol level.

Fish oil, otherwise known as omega-3 fatty acids, can also help improve your blood cholesterol by raising your HDL level. The best dietary sources of fish oil are fatty, deep sea fish such as salmon, mackeral, herring, tuna, anchovies, and sardines. Eating just 3 ounces of fatty fish two or three times a week or taking a single supplemental fish oil capsule daily could have a beneficial effect.

Beta-carotene, vitamin C, and vitamin E can help raise your HDL level. By eating more fruits, vegetables, and whole grains, you will also be eating more of these essential vitamins. Should you take supplements as well? Doctors are divided on the issue. Most would agree, however, that supplements in moderation probably won't hurt and could do a lot of good.

See also Atherosclerosis.

❖ Hives

Hives (urticaria) are small, very itchy, red, swollen bumps on the skin. Hives often appear in clusters; they tend to arise very suddenly and go away just as fast, often within an hour or two. Sometimes, however, hives can last for twenty-four hours or more. Generally, hives are annoying and itchy but not really dangerous. If you get hives in your mouth or throat, however, get medical help at once.

To relieve the itchiness of hives, try placing a cold compress on the affected area. Plain water works well, but you could also soak the compress in cold tea or cold mild herbal teas such as chamomile or red raspberry leaves.

Often hives are an allergic reaction to something you have eaten or a medication you have taken. If you know that particular foods give you hives, avoid them. If a prescription medication you're taking gives you hives, call your doctor at once.

❖ Hypoglycemia

Hypoglycemia occurs when your body doesn't have enough energy-providing glucose in its blood. Symptoms include hunger, fatigue, chills, clammy skin, dizziness, nausea, and a headache. Sometimes your speech is slurred as if you are drunk.

At one time, hypoglycemia was a popular diagnosis, but in fact, it is quite rare except among diabetics. If you have diabetes, you can become hypoglycemic easily, especially if you take too much insulin, skip or postpone meals, or exercise unexpectedly. To treat the symptoms, immediately eat something sugary such as a piece of candy or some sweet fruit juice. Your body needs the sugar, so don't have something that is artificially sweetened. It's important to know what your specific hypoglycemia symptoms usually are so that you can deal with them promptly. Delay can make the problem worse or even lead to coma.

Some diabetics who have frequent episodes of hypoglycemia find that taking supplemental chromium helps them control the problem. There's not much scientific research about the role of chromium in the diet. The daily recommended intake for adults is 50 to 200 micrograms, but some diabetics report that adding 200 micrograms daily, through diet or supplements, helps control their hypoglycemia. If you have diabetes, discuss adding chromium to your diet with your doctor before you try it.

Although some herbs, including dandelion, burdock root, ginseng, and licorice root, are said to help control hypoglycemia in diabetics, there is no evidence that they do. If you have diabetes, do not attempt to treat it with herbs.

If you're not diabetic, the effects of skipping meals or poor nutritional habits may show up as headaches, tiredness, irritability, and depression—symptoms that may be vaguely attributed to low blood sugar. Eating regular, nutritious meals and avoiding caffeine and alcohol will probably provide a miracle cure for your low blood sugar symptoms.

❖ Impotence

Impotence can sometimes affect any man who has had too much to drink, is a substance abuser, is under stress, or is exhausted. However, about ten to twenty million American men are considered impotent—they cannot achieve or maintain an erection long enough to have intercourse on a regular basis. Often the cause is a chronic disease such as alcoholism, diabetes, kidney disease, or atherosclerosis. If you are impotent more than just occasionally, see your doctor. You could have a serious underlying condition.

Over the centuries, hundreds of herbs and other substances (deer antler, for instance) have been recommended as certain cures for impotence. Aside from any placebo effect, these cures are nonsense.

Saw palmetto berries (also called sabal) are used in Germany as a treatment for benign prostate enlargement; some patients there feel this herb also improves their sexual function. However, in the United States saw palmetto is banned. Sarsaparilla (sometimes called smilax) is falsely said to contain the male hormone testosterone. Although sarsaparilla was at one time used to treat syphilis, it is of no use for that or for impotence. Damiana leaves, which come from a shrub found in Mexico, are said to have aphrodisiac qualities when made into a tea or smoked; liqueurs containing damiana are also available. There is no evidence that damiana has any effect at all.

Some herbalists have recently begun recommending gotu kola, an herb from Sri Lanka, or fo-ti, a traditional Chinese herb, as treatments for impotence. However, there is no evidence that either of these is effective. Other completely ineffective herbs for impotence include lovage, vervain, peppermint, ginseng, and savory.

One herb that could actually help impotence is yohimbe, the bark of a tree found in West Africa. Yohimbe is under active scientific scrutiny because alkaloids in the bark do seem to improve erectile function in some men. Although yohimbe is available in Germany, it is not approved for use in the United States. One reason is that yohimbe can have serious side effects, including anxiety, insomnia, hypertension, and nausea.

❖ Indigestion

Indigestion, also sometimes called dyspepsia, is a general term for digestive discomfort such as heartburn, mild nausea, gas, or a bloated or full sensation. Often indigestion is caused by eating fatty or fried foods, very spicy foods, or highly acidic foods.

Several simple herbal remedies for indigestion can relieve symptoms quite effectively. Try some strong, hot peppermint or chamomile tea, or teas made from crushed caraway, anise, or fennel seeds. Ginger or ginseng tea are the traditional Chinese herbal remedies.

See also Gas; Heartburn.

❖ Inflammatory Bowel Disease
See Irritable Bowel Syndrome.

❖ Influenza

Like colds, influenza, or the flu for short, is caused by a virus. Unlike colds, the flu is most common in the winter and early spring and tends to occur in epidemics.

A case of the flu usually starts suddenly and makes you sick quickly. You may have a high fever, chills, muscle aches, sore throat, runny nose, headache, and a cough. You'll probably be sick for several days to a week, and it could take several weeks before you feel completely better. Although influenza is a more serious illness than a common cold, the treatment is very much the same.

Stay home and rest, especially if you have a fever. Don't smoke, and avoid secondhand smoke. Most importantly, drink plenty of fluids—six to eight glasses a day of plain water, fruit juice, mild herbal teas, such as peppermint, linden flowers, red raspberry leaves, or chamomile, chicken broth, uncarbonated soft drinks, and the like. Don't drink alcohol, however.

Some people find that hot, spicy food helps clear their nasal passages, at least temporarily. Gingerroot tea can help temporarily relieve some symptoms, especially upper respiratory congestion. Some people claim that eating garlic or onion at the first hint of illness can ward off the flu; others say that garlic helps relieve flu symptoms, and you will get over it faster. Cooked or raw garlic cloves are equally effective; if you don't like to eat the cloves, try garlic capsules instead.

Echinacea, also sometimes called purple coneflower, is often suggested by herbalists as a way to stimulate your immune system and increase your body's resistance to infection. The usual recommendation is to take echinacea in tincture form (follow the package instructions) at the first sign of flu and to continue taking it while symptoms persist. Although scientists are still uncertain as to exactly how echinacea works, there is no doubt that it can be helpful.

Does vitamin C help prevent or cure the flu? There's not much evidence that it does, but many people swear that taking anywhere from 500 to 1,000 milligrams of supplemental vitamin C a day shortens the duration of the flu and reduces the symptoms. In moderation viatmin C won't hurt and could indeed help, but don't take more than 1,000 milligrams a day. If you get diarrhea, cut back or stop taking the vitamin C.

More than a hundred different viruses can cause a cold, but only a few viruses cause influenza. For that reason, it's possible to make a flu vaccine. If you have heart or respiratory problems, are over age sixty-five, or have a chronic disease such as diabetes, ask your doctor about getting a flu shot.

See also Colds.

❖ Insect Bites

Itchy mosquito bites, painful bee stings, and bites from other annoying bugs can be treated with some simple home herbal remedies.

Bites from mosquitos, chiggers, no-see-ums, and other itch-producing critters often can be relieved simply by rubbing an ice cube on the area. Placing a slice of fresh onion on the bite also often works. Try rubbing chickweed cream, witch hazel, tea tree oil, or lemon balm oil on the bites to relieve itching; poultices made from jewelweed or plantain leaves (plantago) have a similar effect. A cold, wet tea bag, preferably containing green or oolong tea, placed on the bite can also help.

Stings from bees and wasps can be quite painful at first and then itchy later. The first step is to remove the stinger, which may still be embedded in the skin. Using tweezers or a cotton ball, grasp the stinger firmly and pull on it steadily until it is removed. Apply an ice pack or cold-water compress to the sting until the swelling goes down and the pain diminishes. To relieve itching, try the remedies suggested above for mosquito bites.

Some people have severe allergic reactions to bee or wasp stings. The symptoms usually include severe swelling (beyond the immediate area of the sting), intense itching, severe pain, and hives. A severe reaction to a sting is a medical emergency. Get help at once. If you have a minor allergic reaction to a sting, see your doctor; the reaction could be much more severe the next time.

Ticks, such as the large dog tick and the tiny deer tick, give itchy bites that can cause serious illnesses, such as Lyme disease. To remove a tick, soak a cotton ball in rubbing alcohol and rub it over the tick. Grasp the tick firmly as close to the skin as possible and pull on it steadily until it is removed. Alternatively, use tweezers. Wash the area with soap and water. To relieve itching, try the remedies suggested above for mosquito bites.

Various strong-smelling herbal oils are sometimes used on the skin as repellents for mosquitos, ticks, and other biting bugs. Citronella oil, rosemary oil, lavender oil, and myrrh are all traditional favorites. Pennyroyal oil is said to be helpful, especially for mosquitos. However, pennyroyal oil also happens to be highly toxic and can cause coma or even death if taken internally, so stay on the safe side and don't use it. Despite claims, there's no evidence that eating brewer's yeast (or feeding it to your pets) repels mosquitos, fleas, or ticks.

❖ Insomnia

Insomnia—the feeling that you have not slept well or long enough—is the most common sleep complaint. About fifty million adult Americans have trouble getting a good night's sleep. Typically, insomnia is characterized by difficulty falling asleep (taking more than thirty to forty-five minutes), awakening frequently during the nights, or waking up early and being unable to get back to sleep.

Illness, anxiety, stress, indigestion, a headache, some medications (prescription and over-the-counter), jet lag from travel, shift work, and so on can all trigger occasional insomnia. Long-term insomnia (lasting more than three weeks) can be a symptom of serious illness, chronic drug or alcohol abuse, too much caffeine, or depression.

Some simple self-help steps can do a lot for insomnia. Sleep experts agree that the best way to sleep better is keep a regular sleeping schedule. Go to bed about the same time every night, but only if you are tired. Set your alarm to wake you at the same time every morning, even on weekends. If you have a poor night's sleep, get out of bed anyway. Lingering in bed or oversleeping will keep you from establishing a regular biological rhythm.

Alcohol (having a nightcap) may help you sleep at first, but your sleep will probably be fragmented and you will probably wake up in the middle of the night when the alcohol wears off. Don't use alcohol as a remedy for insomnia.

Caffeine or other mild herbal stimulants often cause insomnia. If you're having trouble sleeping, avoid coffee, tea, soda pop, and chocolate for at least six hours before bedtime. Also avoid ginseng tea, maté, and guarana tea.

Some herbs have a sedative effect that can help you get to sleep. Tea made from valerian root is an ancient remedy that is often effective. To make valerian tea, steep 2 teaspoons dried valerian root in 1 cup of boiling water for fifteen minutes. To disguise the tea's pungent taste, try adding a few drops of peppermint oil and a spoonful of honey. If you prefer, try a few drops of valerian root tincture (available at health food stores). Do not use valerian root along with any other sort of prescription or nonprescription sedative drug. Don't use it continually for more than a week.

Hops is another herbal remedy that may help insomnia. Make a strong tea using 2 teaspoons of dried hops in 1 cup of boiling water. Let it steep for five minutes. You could also try hops tincture or capsules. Some herbalists recommend sleeping with a hops-filled pillow.

Passion flower is used in many European herbal formulas for insomnia, although the evidence for its value is slim. In the United States, passion flower is not generally recognized as safe by the Food and Drug Administration.

Drinking a soothing cup of mild herbal tea before bedtime can help you relax and sleep better. Teas made from chamomile, peppermint, catnip, and lemon balm are often recommended by herbalists. Adding 2 or 3 teaspoons of honey to the tea could enhance the relaxation effect.

The amino acid L-tryptophan, while not an herb, is often recommended by herbalists as a sedative. Since 1989, however, when it was linked to twenty-seven deaths and over 5,000 cases of serious illness, L-tryptophan supplements have been banned by the Food and Drug Administration. Taken in small doses of 3 to 5 milligrams at bedtime, the hormone melatonin may be helpful for relieving insomnia from jet lag, night work, and other time-shifts. Supplements can be purchased in health food stores.

❖ Irritable Bowel Syndrome

Crampy pain, gassiness, bloating, diarrhea, and changes in bowel habits are often signs of irritable bowel syndrome (IBS), an ailment that affects at least 10 to 15 percent of all American adults. IBS is second only to the common cold as a cause of missed work days. Irritable bowel syndrome can be severe and can cause a great deal of distress and discomfort, but for many people it is a minor annoyance that can be largely controlled by diet, stress management, and medications prescribed by a physician, when necessary. If you have only occasional and minor IBS symptoms, herbal remedies for constipation, diarrhea, and gas (discussed elsewhere in this book) may be helpful.

In many cases, dietary fiber from bran or other high-fiber foods can help relieve the symptoms of irritable bowel syndrome quite a bit. Add psyllium seeds or other herbal or over-the-counter fiber supplements only after discussing their use with your doctor. At first, you may experience bloating or gas, but as your system gets used to the additional fiber, this should diminish. Be sure to drink six to eight glasses of liquid every day as well—because the fiber needs to absorb water to work.

In the past, IBS was often called colitis or spastic colon, but these terms are no longer used. IBS should not be confused with ulcerative colitis, which is a more serious and sometimes chronic disease.

See also Constipation; Diarrhea; Gas.

❖ Kidney Dialysis
See Dialysis.

❖ Kidney Stones

Pebblelike crystal deposits, commonly known as stones, sometimes form in your kidneys. Most kidney stones remain harmlessly where they are, but sometimes a stone passes from the kidney down through the ureter, a tube that leads to the bladder. This can cause the excruciating, spasmodic pain called renal colic—a condition that accounts for about one million hospitalizations every year, or more than 1 percent of the annual total.

Kidney stones are much more common among men than women, by a ratio of three to one. About 12 to 14 percent of all men experience at least one bout of kidney stone problems by the age of seventy. Those who have had kidney stone trouble once will often develop it again.

About 90 percent of all kidney stones are made of calcium oxalate, so avoiding foods that are high in this mineral can help prevent stone formation. Many strong-tasting greens such as spinach, rhubarb, mustard greens, dandelion greens, Swiss chard, and beet greens are very high in oxalate; so are wheat germ, nuts, and tofu. Beverages such as beer, cocoa, colas, and tea also contain high levels of oxalate.

Numerous herbs with diuretic properties have been recommended over the years for treating the symptoms of kidney stones; the increased urine flow can help you pass the stone naturally. Goldenrod tea can be quite effective for this purpose. Make the flowers into a tea by steeping 2 teaspoonfuls in 2 cups of boiling water. Let it stand for 20 minutes, strain, and drink. Buchu tea, made from the dried leaves of a South African shrub, is popular in Europe; it acts as a mild diuretic and urinary antiseptic. Tea made from parsley leaves also has a useful diuretic effect. For more mild diuretics, try teas made from birch leaves, corn silk, marshmallow, or lovage. Avoid teas made from juniper berries or oil because juniper can have unpredictable and possibly dangerous effects. The herbs gravel root and stone root get their names from their supposed effect on kidney stones, but since they could be toxic, it's a good idea to avoid them. Uva ursi (bearberry) is sometimes recommended for kidney stones. This herb does have useful urinary antiseptic qualities, but it is not an effective diuretic.

A high level of urine production helps keep kidney stones from forming. Drinking six to eight glasses a day of fluids is generally enough to produce a healthy 1 1/2 to 2 1/2 quarts of urine; drink more in hot weather or during times of heavy exertion.

Vitamin B$_6$ deficiency and megadoses of vitamin C over 2,000 milligrams a day have been linked to kidney stone formation. If you have ever had a kidney stone, discuss any vitamin therapy with your doctor before trying it.

❖ Liver Disease

See Alcoholism; Gallstones; Hepatitis.

❖ Lupus Erythematosus

Lupus erythematosus is a chronic autoimmune disease that causes inflammation of various parts of the body, especially the skin, joints, blood vessels, and kidneys. Between 1.4 and 2 million Americans have been diagnosed with lupus—more than have AIDS, cerebral palsy, multiple sclerosis, sickle cell anemia, and cystic fibrosis combined. Lupus affects 1 out of every 185 Americans; it occurs ten to fifteen times more often among women than men. For most people, lupus is a mild disease affecting only a few organs, but for others, the disease is more severe and even life-threatening.

One type of lupus, called discoid lupus, is limited only to the skin. Patients get a red rash on the face, neck, and scalp. Systemic lupus is usually more severe than discoid lupus and can affect almost any organ or system of the body. The most common symptoms include achy or swollen joints, fever, prolonged fatigue, skin rashes, anemia, kidney problems, pleurisy, and sensitivity to sunlight.

In many cases, lupus symptoms can be controlled with anti-inflammatory drugs and patients can lead fairly normal lives. Lupus patients should be very careful about trying any herbal remedies for lupus symptoms or those of any other illness. Alfalfa, for example, contains the amino acid L-canavanine, which can worsen lupus symptoms. Herbs such as angelica, dong quai (a traditional Chinese herb), parsley, and St. John's wort can worsen the problem of sun sensitivity.

The omega-3 fatty acids found in fish oils seem to show promise as a way to help control lupus symptoms. Studies have shown that high doses of omega-3 in the form of capsules can help reduce lupus joint inflammation, although no more than aspirin does, and at a much higher cost.

Many lupus patients report that their symptoms of sun sensitivity and inflamed skin are reduced when they take vitamin E in doses of 800 to 2,000 IU daily. If you have lupus, discuss taking supplemental vitamin E with your doctor before trying it.

❖ Macular Degeneration

The macula is the central, most sensitive part of the retina in your eye. Age-related macular degeneration is a blinding eye disease that affects this small but crucial area. It destroys the sharp vision needed for seeing objects clearly and for common daily activities such as driving and reading. Fortunately, macular degeneration almost never results in complete blindness, since side vision is usually not affected.

The greatest risk factor for macular degeneration is simply age. The problem is rare among people under the age of sixty. Among people age seventy-five and older, the risk of macular degeneration is 30 percent. If you have high blood pressure, diabetes, or cardiovascular disease, you are more likely to develop macular degeneration. Women get macular degeneration more often than men. If you are white, you are much more likely to have macular degeneration than if you are African-American. Smoking may also increase your risk.

Sadly, little can be done to help macular degeneration, so prevention may be the best approach. The anthocyanosides found in dried blueberries (also called bilberries) may help prevent eye problems, including macular degeneration. The concentration required, however, is far greater than could be obtained simply by eating the berries or drinking a tea made from them. A commercial bilberry extract that claims to be high in anthocyanosides is available at heath food stores. Discuss the use of anthocyanoside extract with your doctor before trying it. Solid evidence indicates that people who eat food high in carotenoids (the orange or yellow pigments found naturally in such foods as carrots, squash, and sweet potatoes) have a 43 percent lower risk of developing macular degeneration. Two carotenoids—lutein and zeaxanthin—have been shown to be particularly effective. It's possible that the carotenoids are similar to natural yellowish pigments that are lost from the retina when macular degeneration occurs. However, taking supplemental vitamin A, vitamin E, and vitamin C seems to have no effect on reducing the risk—you have to eat your vegetables to get the benefits.

Herbs that are traditionally recommended for vision problems—eyebright, goldenseal, yellow dock, and others—have no effect on macular degeneration. Don't use them.

See also Cataracts; Glaucoma.

❖ Menopause

A woman's reproductive life comes to a natural end as she reaches middle age. Her menstrual cycles gradually cease as her ovaries reduce production of the female hormones estrogen and progesterone. Menopause generally occurs between the ages of forty and fifty-five; the average age is fifty-one. When a woman has not had a menstrual period for a year, her body is producing only 10 percent of the estrogen and virtually none of the progesterone it made before menopause.

Although every woman experiences menopause differently, each is likely to go through some physical and emotional changes as a result of the hormonal loss. Modern medicine, especially hormone replacement therapy, can help relieve most menopause problems. Some herbal remedies may also help some of the minor symptoms.

Hot Flashes

Probably the most common symptom of menopause is the hot flash. Over 75 percent of all menopausal women will get them. Hot flashes are often described as a sudden wave of heat, causing flushing on the face and neck. The flashes can last anywhere from a few seconds to an hour, although most last just a minute or two. They often occur at night and disrupt your sleep, leading to insomnia and fatigue. Although scientists still don't know exactly why hot flashes occur, they do know that estrogen supplements are very helpful for reducing or eliminating them. The traditional Chinese herb dong quai and the South American herb gotu kola are both said to help hot flashes. These herbs have probably been falsely credited for the natural cessation of the hot flashes, which usually stop after a year or so.

Vaginal Dryness

When estrogen levels drop during menopause, the lining of the vagina becomes thinner, drier, and less elastic. These changes can cause discomfort during intercourse and can also contribute to vaginal and urinary tract infections. Estrogen replacement therapy can be helpful for relieving vaginal dryness. Water-based vaginal lubricants, sold over the counter in any drugstore, are very effective. Avoid oil-based lubricants, since these can lead to infection. Do not use the oily contents of vitamin E capsules.

Osteoporosis

A serious consequence of menopause can be osteoporosis, or thin, brittle bones caused by a loss of bone mass. After the age of about thirty-five, women begin to lose more bone than their bodies produce. For about six to eight years after menopause, the decrease in bone mass occurs even faster. The result can be bones that break easily, causing crippling injuries that can lead to death. (See the section on Osteoporosis for more information on this preventable problem.)

To prevent osteoporosis later, increase your calcium intake now. Most doctors recommend 1,000 to 1,200 milligrams of calcium daily for younger women and 1,500 milligrams a day for postmenopausal women. For your body to use calcium properly, you also need adequate levels of vitamin D. Your body produces most its own vitamin D from exposure to sunlight; you also get some from your diet. As you age, your body's ability to make its own vitamin D is reduced, so it's especially important for menopausal women to get the recommended 400 IU a day. Discuss your calcium needs with your doctor. Supplemental calcium and vitamin D may be needed. Also discuss estrogen replacement therapy with your doctor. Recent studies have proven that women who begin taking estrogen within five years of menopause and continue it for the rest of their lives have a substantially lower risk of bone fractures, including broken hips.

Phytoestrogens

Women who regularly eat soy products such as tofu and soy milk report fewer and less severe menopause symptoms.

This is probably because soybeans contain large amounts of phytoestrogens, plant estrogens that are similar to human estrogen. Phytoestrogens are found at lower concentrations in other plant foods such as cabbage, garlic, oats, sesame seeds, and flax seeds. Black cohosh, an herb traditionally used by Native Americans for menopausal symptoms, does contain some phytoestrogens and is often recommended in Europe. Licorice root, hops, sage, and ginseng are said to help stimulate estrogen production, although little evidence supports this. (Avoid licorice root if you have high blood pressure or any sort of heart condition.) Saw palmetto (sabal), an herb used in Europe but banned by the U.S. Food and Drug Administration, may also contain phytoestrogens. However, none of these foods or herbs contain enough of any estrogenlike compounds to be used as substitutes for estrogen replacement therapy.

Other herbs sometimes suggested for general menopause symptoms include damiana, red raspberry leaves, chaste tree berries, alfalfa, motherwort, nettle, St. John's wort, and dandelion root. None contain any sort of phytoestrogen or estrogen-stimulating compounds and none are helpful for menopausal symptoms.

See also Osteoporosis; Urinary Tract Infections.

❖ Menstrual Cramps

During menstruation, the lining of a woman's uterus produces hormones called prostaglandins, which help the uterus contract and expel its lining. Those same contractions, however, also produce the discomfort of menstrual cramps. Most women experience at least some mild cramping with every period.

Numerous traditional herbs are recommended for menstrual cramps. In traditional European herbal medicine, raspberry leaf tea, lovage, peppermint tea, chaste tree berries, motherwort, calendula, sage, yarrow, rue, parsley, rosemary, tansy, chamomile, St. John's wort, and valerian root are all considered helpful. Ginseng, dong quai, and dan shen (sage root) are suggested in traditional Chinese herbal medicine. Native Americans used cramp bark, lobelia, blue cohosh root, and black cohosh root. Many herbalists today often suggest evening primrose oil. Do any of these herbal remedies work? Black cohosh root (also called snakeroot) is popular in Europe; many women claim it is helpful, but there is no real information on its value and safety. Blue cohosh root (also sometimes called squaw root) is often recommended by herbalists as an emmenagogue, a menstrual flow stimulator. However, the root contains numerous alkaline substances that could be dangerous. Likewise, the traditional Native American herb life root or squaw weed contains alkaloids toxic to the liver. Do not use it for menstrual discomfort or anything else. Despite claims, there's little evidence that gamma-linolenic acid (GLA), the active ingredient in evening primrose oil (and also borage seed oil) helps menstrual cramps.

Many of the herbs traditionally recommended, such as lovage, parsley, goldenrod, and dandelion root, act as mild diuretics, which can help relieve cramping. Others, such as ginseng (and also tea and coffee), act as mild stimulants, which can also help relieve cramping. Most of the other remedies don't really contain anything that has been proven to help. Herbal menstrual remedies usually are taken as teas or infusions, however, so it's possible that the relaxing effect of preparing and drinking a hot beverage does help relieve cramps. Do any herbal remedies work as well as simply taking an over-the-counter nonsteroidal anti-inflammatory drug such as ibuprofen? Probably not.

Some herbs, such as angelica, gentian, rosemary, rue, tansy, blue cohosh, and black cohosh, are sometimes recommended as emmenagogues, or herbs that stimulate the menstrual flow. In many old herbals, however, emmenagogue is a euphemism for abortifacients, or herbs that promote miscarriages. If your menstrual period is late, do not attempt to start it by using herbs since you could be pregnant. Taking herbal medications during the early stages of pregnancy could harm your unborn baby. Attempting to induce a miscarriage with herbs or in any other way is dangerous and possibly fatal. See your doctor if your period is late or you think you are pregnant.

Some herbs that contain high amounts of calcium or magnesium may help reduce menstrual cramping. Calcium and magnesium help your body regulate muscle tone; too little can lead to cramps. Good herbal or natural sources of calcium include alfalfa, bee pollen, chamomile tea, dandelion leaves, fennel, garlic, ginseng, kelp, and watercress. Good herbal or natural sources of magnesium include bee pollen, dandelion leaves, garlic, red clover flowers, wheat germ, and brewer's yeast. Try taking these herbs in the days just before and during your period.

See also Premenstrual Syndrome (PMS).

❖ Migraine

The severe pain of a migraine headache is usually felt on just one side of your head. The pain is often accompanied by a range of other unpleasant symptoms, such as nausea, vomiting, aversion to light, and cold hands and feet. A typical migraine lasts for about six hours. Warning signs, called the prodrome or aura, often start an hour or two before the headache strikes. The warning signs are usually visual—many people see flashing lights or zigzag patterns. Only about 20 to 30 percent of all migraine headaches begin with an aura, however. Migraines are a fairly common type of headache—some sixteen to eighteen million Americans, seventy percent of them women, get them.

Researchers don't fully understand the causes of a migraine. They suspect that your levels of a substance called serotonin, which your body produces to help regulate the diameter of blood vessels, play an important role. Serotonin levels may fluctuate as a result of stress, low blood sugar, or changes in your estrogen level. If the level changes too much, a migraine could result. In addition, foods, especially those that naturally contain a substance called amine, can trigger a migraine. This is because amines can dilate your blood vessels.

Amines of various sorts are found in many foods. Tyramine, for example, is found in many nuts and seeds and in alcohol; phenylethylamine is found in chocolate. Other foods that contain amines include most beans and legumes and many fruits. Aged, pickled, preserved, fermented, cured, or cultured foods can also be migraine triggers. Avoid alcoholic beverages, beer, and wine, pickles, cultured dairy products such as sour cream and buttermilk, and baked goods containing yeast, if you are susceptible. Nitrites, nitrates, and monosodium glutamate (MSG), chemicals often added to processed foods, can also trigger migraine headaches. Caffeine can be another migraine trigger. Most doctors recommend limiting your caffeine intake if you get migraines.

Some herbal remedies can provide relief from a migraine headache. Ginger has been used as a migraine treatment in traditional Chinese medicine for centuries. If you eat a small piece of fresh gingerroot at the first hint of a migraine, you could forestall the headache. An old European remedy is to lie down and rub a few drops of lavender oil into your temples when you feel a migraine coming. This does seem to forestall the headache for some people. Some recent research suggests that fish oil capsules could help relieve and prevent migraines. In one study, patients who regularly took fish oil capsules had fewer and less severe migraines. Herbalists say that ginkgo biloba extract can help because it improves cerebral circulation. In theory, this should make your migraine worse, but some patients claim ginkgo works for them. The sedative effect of valerian root tea can be mildly helpful if you have a migraine. Echinacea is sometimes recommended for migraines, but it probably has little, if any, effect. The herbs mullein, peppermint, rosemary, and lovage are also sometimes suggested, but they too, are ineffective.

An herb that is under active investigation for its beneficial effects on migraine headaches is feverfew. The leaves of this plant contain a substance that relaxes the blood vessels in your brain. Patients who eat a few fresh leaves or take an extract of the leaves every day have fewer and less severe migraines. It is possible to buy feverfew tablets and extracts at health food stores, but consumers need to be very cautious. Many of these products contain little of the active ingredient. Although feverfew shows promise as a migraine treatment, discuss it with your doctor before trying it.

See also Headaches.

❖ Morning Sickness

Almost all women have some morning sickness—nausea and vomiting—during the first three months of pregnancy. Fortunately, there are some useful steps you can take to relieve the symptoms. Many women find that eating plain, unsalted crackers the moment they awaken in the morning—even before getting out of bed—can help quite a bit. Others find that eating small, frequent meals throughout the day instead of three larger meals is helpful. In general, avoid spicy, greasy, and strong-smelling foods. Some women find that ginger, in the form of capsules, tea, or fresh root, helps relieve nausea.

Vomiting can cause dehydration if you don't drink enough liquids to replace the fluid you lose. Avoid coffee and other caffeine-containing beverages; also avoid carbonated soft drinks. Instead, drink plain water, broth, unsweetened fruit juice, or mild herbal teas such as peppermint, lemon balm, or chamomile. Avoid all alcoholic beverages during pregnancy.

Raspberry leaf tea is often recommended as a safe and enjoyable herbal drink during pregnancy. It is said to help relieve morning sickness. If you want to try raspberry leaf tea, be sure to purchase exactly that at the health food store. Take care not to purchase raspberry-flavored black tea by mistake.

See also Pregnancy.

❖ Motion Sickness

Nausea and vomiting as a result of constant, unpredictable movement, better known as motion sickness, is very common. Car sickness, sea sickness, and air sickness are all variations on this basic theme. Motion sickness may be nearly inevitable in some circumstances—a boat trip in rough weather, for example. In most cases, however, there are some steps you can take to reduce or eliminate the symptoms. Eat a small, simple meal before the trip begins. If you must eat while traveling, stick to simple carbohydrates such as plain crackers, rolls, potatoes, and rice; fruits such as apples and bananas are usually easy to keep down. Avoid caffeine, carbonated beverages, acidic fruit juices, and any sort of alcoholic beverage; instead, stick to plain water or mild herbal teas, such as peppermint or chamomile.

There are any number of folk remedies for motion sickness. Sucking on a slice of lemon, eating some olives, or chewing on fresh peppermint leaves (or drinking strong peppermint tea) are typical recommendations. Pennyroyal oil, made from an herb closely related to peppermint, is sometimes recommended, but this toxic oil should not be taken internally.

An herbal remedy that is often very effective is ginger. It seems to work best if taken about twenty minutes before the trip begins. The form of the ginger doesn't seem to matter much. Try swallowing 1/2 teaspoon of ground ginger (mixed in water or placed in a gelatin capsule), eating a small piece of fresh gingerroot, having a cup of gingerroot tea, or eating a few pieces of candied ginger. Don't overdo it, however. Too much ginger can cause mouth and intestinal irritation.

❖ Mouth Sores

Mouth sores on the inside linings of the lips, cheeks, or tongue are a painful nuisance for many people. Recurrent mouth sores, known medically as aphthous stomatitis and popularly as oral ulcers or canker sores, afflict about 20 percent of the population.

What causes mouth sores is not well understood. They don't seem to be caused by a virus or bacteria, and they're not contagious. In some cases, they may be symptomatic of an allergic reaction to certain foods or related to hormonal changes during the menstrual cycle. Mouth sores are often caused by an injury to the lining of your mouth, such as biting the inside of your cheek or having poorly fitting dentures. If a dental problem, such as a broken tooth, is causing your mouth sores, see your dentist soon.

To relieve the discomfort of mouth sores, avoid spicy or acidic foods and drink. Avoid commercial mouthwashes, but do try rinsing your mouth with warm, salty water several times a day. Astringent herbs such as goldenseal, vervain, calendula, raspberry leaves, rosemary, and sage are often recommended for mouth sores. Myrrh, which has a very strong taste, is also sometimes suggested. They can be made into strong teas for rinsing the mouth several times a day. Some herbalists suggest adding a few drops of echinacea tincture to the tea for an added antibiotic effect.

❖ Multiple Sclerosis

Multiple sclerosis (MS) is a chronic disease of the central nervous system that interferes to varying degrees with speech, walking, and other basic functions. The symptoms of

MS occur when, for unknown reasons, the fatty sheath that forms a covering for the nerve fibers of the central nervous system is destroyed. This causes the impulses that travel along the nerve to be disrupted, much as removing the insulation from around an electrical wire causes interference with the transmission of signals. MS symptoms can run the gamut from slight blurring of vision to complete paralysis, but the majority of people with MS do not become severely disabled and continue to lead productive and satisfying lives. About 350,000 Americans have MS, with nearly 200 new cases diagnosed every week. Multiple sclerosis often strikes people in their prime, most commonly between the ages of twenty and forty. Nearly twice as many women as men have MS.

The symptoms of MS vary greatly, depending upon where the nerve damage occurs. Typically, someone with multiple sclerosis has periods of active disease, called exacerbations, and symptom-free periods, called remissions. There is no cure for multiple sclerosis. Physicians can only treat the symptoms.

Some preliminary evidence shows that the gamma-linolenic acid (GLA) in evening primrose oil has a beneficial effect on multiple sclerosis, possibly slowing its progression in some patients. However, of all the other numerous special diets, herb formulas, and food or vitamin supplements that claim to miraculously cure or help multiple sclerosis, none so far have been found to have genuine therapeutic value. If any of these seem to help a few people, at least for a time, it is probably because MS is an episodic disease with naturally occurring remissions. Neither the Swank diet nor the MacDougal diet have been accepted by the National MS Society's Medical Advisory Board as being effective, but these diets are not harmful. The Swank diet, for example, is basically just an extremely low-fat diet, while the MacDougal diet combines a low-fat approach with a gluten-free diet and supplemental vitamins and minerals. Some other nutritional approaches that claim to be therapeutic, however, are based on unproven theories that have never been tested in controlled studies. The same is true of therapies based on megadoses of vitamins or minerals. For example, injections of vitamin B_{12} will not benefit MS patients, because there is no evidence that the disease is caused by vitamin B_{12} deficiency. Treatment with massive doses of vitamin C (sometimes called megascorbic therapy or orthomolecular therapy) is not only ineffective and possibly dangerous, it is also very expensive.

❖ Muscle Pain

Almost everyone occasionally experiences sore or aching muscles after overdoing an activity or exercise. As a rule, the discomfort gradually goes away over a few days, but there are some useful herbal remedies that can relieve the aches in the meantime.

Arnica is an old herbal standby that can be quite effective for relieving muscle pain. It seems to work best in tincture form, but arnica ointments are also helpful. Rub the arnica preparation into the skin above the affected area. Although calendula and comfrey ointments are also sometimes suggested, they are not very effective.

Wintergreen oil (also called menthol) is an ingredient in many nonprescription ointments for aching muscles. It's what gives them their distinctive aroma. Mint oils, including wintergreen, peppermint, and pennyroyal, are all sometimes suggested as treatments for sore muscles. Pennyroyal oil is very toxic if taken internally, so stay on the safe side and use another herb with the same effect. Other oils that may be helpful include St. John's wort, thyme, lavender, and juniper. Rub a few drops of the oil into the skin at the affected area. Since the temporary relief probably comes from the counterirritating effect of the oils, never use rubbing oils on broken skin, and stop using them if a rash or irritation develops. Never take any of these oils internally.

Hot baths often help relax sore muscles. Try adding some rosemary or thyme leaves to the bathwater—they smell nice and are said to help soothe aches.

❖ Nail Health

Like your hair, your nails are made of dead, hardened protein called keratin that is actually quite similar to the surface layer of your skin. Nail problems, like skin problems, are often painful and unsightly, but they are usually not particularly dangerous.

For good nail health, doctors generally recommend a well-balanced, nutritious diet along with a daily multivitamin supplement. If you're still having nail problems a few months after improving your diet, try adding additional vitamin E (200 IU daily) and fish oil (1,000 milligrams daily). You could also try adding the nutrient biotin to your diet. Brewer's yeast, egg yolks, alfalfa, burdock root, dandelion leaves, kelp, soybeans, and bananas are good sources of this B-complex vitamin. Some doctors feel that the mineral silica is important for good nail health. Alfalfa and horsetail are naturally high in this mineral.

❖ Nausea

Nausea, that unpleasant abdominal feeling of queasiness or being on the verge of vomiting, can have many causes. Morning sickness, motion sickness, chemotherapy for cancer, hangover, indigestion, and minor intestinal illnesses are all possible culprits.

In many cases, mild nausea can be relieved by eating small amounts of plain, bland foods such as saltine crackers, toast, white rice, and fruits such as apples and bananas. Sometimes hot chicken broth helps. Avoid caffeine, carbonated beverages, acidic fruit juices, and any sort of alcoholic beverage.

An old folk remedy for nausea that sometimes helps is to suck on a slice of lemon. Strong peppermint or chamomile tea can be effective for relieving nausea. Pennyroyal oil, made from an herb closely related to peppermint, is sometimes recommended, but this toxic oil should not be taken internally.

An herbal remedy for nausea that is often very effective is ginger. Try swallowing 1/2 teaspoon of ground ginger (mixed in water or placed in a gelatin capsule), eating a small piece of fresh gingerroot, having a cup of gingerroot tea, or eating a few pieces of candied ginger. Even flat ginger ale can help. Don't overdo, however. Too much ginger can cause mouth and intestinal irritation.

Persistent nausea or vomiting could be a sign of a more serious problem, such as an ulcer. See your doctor if your nausea is very severe, doesn't go away in a few days, or is accompanied by abdominal pain.

See also Chemotherapy; Hangover; Indigestion; Morning Sickness; Motion Sickness.

❖ Obesity

Nearly half the American population is overweight or obese, which explains why at any given time, one out of every six Americans is on a weight-loss diet. Obesity (weighing 20 percent or more over your desirable weight) has numerous serious health consequences. Cancers of the breast, uterus, and ovaries are more common in obese women; cancers of the colon, rectum, and prostate are more common in obese men. People who are overweight or obese are much more likely to develop adult-onset diabetes, heart disease, respiratory problems, arthritis, gallbladder disease, and menstrual problems.

Determining what the right weight is for you depends to some degree on your body type and age. Some recent research suggests, for example, that most people can get a little heavier as they grow older without added risk to their health while other research contradicts this. The chart below gives suggested weight ranges for adults based on studies by the National Research Council of the National Academy of Sciences. If your weight for your height falls within the guidelines of the chart, you probably are at or near a healthy weight for you.

Suggested Weights for Adults

Height	Weight in Pounds	
	19–34 Years	*35 Years and Older*
5'0"	97–128	108–138
5'1"	101–132	111–143
5'2"	104–137	115–148
5'3"	107–141	119–152
5'4"	111–146	122–157
5'5"	114–150	126–162
5'6"	118–155	130–167
5'7"	121–160	134–172
5'8"	125–164	138–178
5'9"	129–169	142–183
5'10"	132–174	146–188
5'11"	136–179	151–194
6'0"	140–184	155–199
6'1"	144–189	159–205
6'2"	148–195	164–210
6'3"	152–200	168–216
6'4"	156–205	173–222

Note: Assumes height without shoes and weight without clothes. The higher weights in the ranges generally apply to men, who tend to have larger muscles and bones; the lower weights generally apply to women, who tend to have smaller muscles and bones.

The best way to lose weight is eat less and exercise more. There are no magic powders, pills, or other potions that lead to magical weight loss without dieting and exercise. Crash diets that promise that you will lose ten pounds in one week, fad diets that restrict you to certain foods, and very low-calorie diets that allow only liquid nutrition may indeed lead to temporary, short-term weight loss. These diets inevitably fail in the long run and may even be dangerous to your heath. Yo-yo dieting, where you rapidly lose weight and just as rapidly gain it back, simply makes it even harder to lose weight later. In the end, large fluctuations in weight may be more detrimental to your health than remaining overweight. A far better approach is to permanently modify your eating habits and get more exercise. Long-term, permanent weight loss is a slow but steady process. Most doctors agree that losing just a pound a week is a realistic goal.

Many herbs and other dietary supplements, either alone or in combination, have been recommended as aids to losing weight. No herb or herbal formula burns fat away, lets you lose weight while you sleep, guarantees that you will never feel hungry, or causes you to lose weight in any other magical way. Be very wary of full-page magazines ads that offer a secret herbal or scientific formula for weight loss.

Spirulina, a form of green algae, is sometimes recommended by herbalists and natural medicine practitioners as a way to lose weight quickly. Taking an expensive, 500-milligram spirulina tablet with each meal will supposedly control your appetite, suppress hunger pangs, and help you eat less. The scientific basis for the efficacy of spirulina is said to be the amino acid L-phenylalanine, which is believed to have an influence on the brain's appetite control center. This claim was carefully reviewed by the Food and Drug Administration in 1979 and found to be baseless. Similarly, juices made from alfalfa, barley grass, or wheat grass are said to help dieters lose weight. Although the fresh juices may be a good source of vitamins and minerals, there is nothing in them that melts away fat.

The traditional Chinese herb ma huang (also called ephedra) is sometimes recommended for weight loss, usually as a tea. Ma huang contains ephedrine, which can be useful for the treatment of asthma, but does little to help you lose weight. In fact, because ma huang can also raise your blood pressure and increase your heart rate, among other undesirable side effects, using it to lose weight could actually be dangerous. Do not use ma huang for any reason if you have high blood pressure, a heart condition, diabetes, or thyroid disease.

Bladderwrack, kelp, and other seaweeds taken as teas, tinctures, or in capsules are said to help stimulate slow metabolisms, which in turn leads to weight loss. The stimulation supposedly occurs because iodine in the seaweed causes your body to produce additional thyroid hormones. In fact, this would only work if you happened to have a thyroid deficiency due to lack of iodine, and such a deficiency is extremely unlikely because of the near universal use of iodized salt. Even if seaweed did stimulate the production of thyroid hormones, this would be a potentially dangerous way to lose weight. Bladderwrack and kelp are very similar—indeed, some scientists say identical—seaweeds. Perhaps to make their products seem more impressive, producers of weight-loss herbal mixtures often call these seaweeds by their scientific names, *Fucus vesiculosis*.

Many so-called slimming teas or weight-loss teas contain herbs that act as diuretics. That is, they stimulate your kidneys to produce more urine. This is turn can cause quick weight loss, often of several pounds, in just a few days. Among the herbs often used are dandelion root, parsley, lovage, corn silk, black cohosh, wood betony, goldenrod, and bearberry (uva ursi). Buchu tea, made from the dried leaves of a South African shrub, is popular in Europe as a weight-loss tea. The weight you lose in this artificial way won't be permanently gone. You will gain it back as soon as you stop taking the diuretic. Using diuretics to lose weight can be dangerous, particularly if you have any other medical condition, such as diabetes or high blood pressure. When you pass more urine, you deplete your body of essential minerals, particularly potassium and sodium. If you take herbal diuretics for more than a few days, you could seriously disturb your body's mineral balance, with possibly fatal consequences.

Amino acid supplements are another spurious approach to weight loss. The amino acids L-carnitine, L-tyrosine, L-ornithine, L-phenylalanine, and L-tryptophan are all said to aid in weight control. For example, L-ornithine is misleadingly said to metabolize excess body fat. Large doses of single amino acids are unlikely to have any effect, however, and could be harmful. The Food and Drug Administration does not consider single amino acid supplements to be generally recognized as safe. In addition, since 1989, the FDA has banned sales of products that consist mostly or entirely of the amino acid L-tryptophan.

The mineral chromium picolinate is sometimes recommended by natural medicine practitioners as a supplement to help speed weight loss. It is often combined in capsules with herbs such as ma huang (discussed above) and labeled as a "thermogenic" or "fat-burning" formula. The capsules are sold at high cost in health-food stores. Supposedly, these capsules will make you lose weight without reducing your caloric intake. This magical result is said to occur because chromium picolinate reduces insulin resistance, which makes your body burn glucose instead of turning it into fat. The science behind all this is preliminary and speculative, but it is certain that you cannot lose weight simply by adding chromium picolinate to your diet.

In general, a good weight-loss diet is the same as a good, healthy diet for anyone: high in fiber, low in fat, with lots of fresh fruits, fresh vegetables, and whole grains.

❖ Osteoporosis

Osteoporosis, a loss of bone mass that results in thin, brittle bones that fracture easily, is the leading cause of bone fractures in postmenopausal women and the elderly. Over 1.3 million osteoporosis-related fractures occur each year in the United States, primarily of the hip, spine, and wrist. The cost to society is estimated at $7 to $10 billion.

Osteoporosis can't be cured, but it can be prevented or slowed down by making sure you include enough calcium in your diet. Calcium is essential for building and maintaining strong bones—your body contains about three pounds of it. According to the National Institutes of Health, only half the children and young adults in America are getting their optimal calcium intake, which is between 1,200 and 1,500 milligrams a day. By some other estimates, eight out of ten American women don't get enough calcium. The NIH now recommends that women age twenty-five to fifty and men age twenty-five to sixty-five get 1,000 milligrams of calcium daily. (In addition to helping prevent osteoporosis, there is some evidence that this level of calcium may also protect against high blood pressure.)

Menopausal women are at particular risk of osteoporosis. This is because their decreased estrogen levels cause bone loss to be accelerated for a period of about six to eight years; after that, bone loss becomes more gradual. To lower the risk, doctors now recommend that menopausal women get 1,000 to 1,500 milligrams of calcium daily. Both men and women over the age of sixty-five should aim for 1,500 milligrams daily.

The best way to get enough calcium is through diet. Milk is the best dietary source of calcium: one 8-ounce glass of nonfat milk has about 300 milligrams of calcium. Some herbs such as alfalfa, dandelion leaves, fennel, chamomile, horsetail, kelp, and watercress contain calcium. However, consuming these herbs would meet your daily requirement only if you ate them in very large amounts. Add more calcium to your diet by including calcium-rich foods or some of the new calcium-fortified fruit juices, cereals, and breads.

To be certain of getting enough calcium, especially if you are pregnant or nursing or if you are menopausal, discuss taking a calcium supplement with your doctor. Most daily multivitamin supplements include about half the daily calcium recommendation. Menopausal women should also discuss estrogen replacement therapy, since this has been shown to significantly reduce the risk of fractures.

Certain drugs, such as aluminum antacids, cortisone, thyroxine, and some antibiotics, may accelerate bone loss. If you need to take drugs of this sort for an extended time, discuss calcium supplements with your doctor.

For your body to use calcium properly, you also need to have adequate levels of vitamin D. Your body produces its own vitamin D from exposure to sunlight and also gets it from your diet. As you age, your body's ability to make its own vitamin D is reduced, so it's especially important for you to get the recommended 400 IU a day.

Tobacco, alcohol, and caffeine can interfere with your body's absorption of calcium. Cut back on alcohol and caffeine. If you smoke, stop. Even if you increase your calcium intake, your chances of osteoporosis remain high if you continue to smoke.

Inactivity is another risk factor for osteoporosis, so remain active as you get older. Weight-bearing exercise, such as walking, jogging, and bike riding, is very helpful for building bone strength and preventing osteoporosis. A brisk daily walk for only twenty to thirty minutes can be very beneficial. It will help keep your bones strong and probably will make you feel better in general.

See also Menopause.

❖ Parkinson's Disease

Parkinson's disease is a slowly progressive disease that causes tremors or trembling of the arms and legs, stiffness and rigidity of the muscles, and slowness of movement. Parkinson's disease (PD) affects more than one million Americans. By some estimates, 1 percent of the population over age sixty has PD and each year some 50,000 new cases are diagnosed. The cause of Parkinson's disease is unknown, although researchers believe that it is related to a chemical imbalance in the brain. There is no cure for Parkinson's disease, but many patients respond well to drugs and physical therapy.

The brains of Parkinson's patients no longer produce a vital neurotransmitter substance called dopamine. Levodopa, more commonly known as L-dopa, is the primary drug for treating Parkinson's disease. In combination with another drug, carbidopa (Sinemet is the brand name), L-dopa helps replace some of the missing dopamine and relieves Parkinson's symptoms.

Research over the years has shown that the diet of Parkinson's patients has a lot to do with how well they respond to L-dopa. Today, most doctors recommend that Parkinson's patients eat a protein-restricted diet, because digesting protein releases amino acids, including L-tyrosine, into the bloodstream. These amino acids then compete with the L-dopa to cross into the brain. The more amino acids in the blood, the less L-dopa gets into the brain, and the less effective the medication will be.

The amino acid L-tyrosine can have a similar effect as the medicine L-dopa. Research into the value of L-tyrosine as an alternative treatment for Parkinson's disease is now in progress, but little is known about the effects of using high doses over a long period, and PD patients often live with their condition for twenty years. Although L-tyrosine supplements are available at health food stores, do not attempt to treat your Parkinson's disease symptoms with them. The Food and Drug Administration has not approved L-tyrosine as a drug.

There is no evidence that Parkinson's disease has anything to do with nutritional deficiencies, and there is no evidence that any particular vitamins or minerals help the condition. You may want to take a daily multivitamin supplement, but megadoses of vitamins do not help Parkinson's disease and could be dangerous. High doses of vitamin A and vitamin E, for example, can be toxic.

Herbal remedies are sometimes recommended for conditions that accompany Parkinson's disease, such as excess salivation or constipation. If you wish to try an herbal remedy for anything related to your PD, discuss it with your doctor first.

❖ Poison Ivy

The bane of hikers, gardeners, and anyone else who spends time outdoors, poison ivy contains an irritating oil that causes an itchy, oozing rash when it comes in contact with your skin. Only about half of all people who touch poison ivy, poison oak, or poison sumac will have the allergic reaction that causes the rash, but you won't know which group you are in until it happens to you. Even worse, you can lose your immunity without warning.

Whether or not you know you are allergic, learning to recognize and avoid these plants is a good idea. Poison ivy shrubs and vines are widely found throughout the United States and Canada. An old adage for avoiding it is, "Leaves of three, let it be." The plant has green, lobe-shaped leaves arranged in clusters of three to a stalk. In the autumn, the leaves turn bright red and small white berries are also present. Poison oak plants are bushy and have serrated leaves that resemble oak leaves; the leaves also grow in clusters of three. Poison sumac is a woody shrub found mostly in the southeastern United States. The leaflets grow in pairs along a stalk.

All parts of poison ivy, poison oak, and poison sumac—not just the leaves—can cause nasty rashes. Even dead plants still contain the irritating oil. You don't have to touch the plant directly to develop the rash. The oil could get on your shoes, for example, and rub off on your hands hours later when you remove the shoes. Cats and dogs sometimes wander through poison ivy patches and get the oil on their fur; it can then come off on you when you touch the animal.

If you know you have been in contact with an irritating plant, wash the affected area with strong soap and water within fifteen to thirty minutes of exposure. Be sure to scrub under your fingernails if you think you may have touched the plant with your hands. Washing can sometimes forestall the rash or reduce its severity. If you can't wash right away, do it as soon as you can. Clothing, shoes, and anything else that has been in contact with the plant should also be thoroughly washed. Sometimes you don't realize that you have poison ivy until a day or two later. In that case, wash everything that has touched your skin in the previous few days, including bedding, the steering wheel of your car, and so on.

The intense itching, redness, blisters, streaking, and oozing of a rash from poison ivy, poison oak, or poison sumac usually appears within twelve to forty-eight hours after contact with the plant. The rash can appear anywhere on the body, but it usually appears on the face, neck, arms, hands, legs, and feet; its severity will depend on how sensitive you are to the irritating oil. The rash may spread to other parts of your body over the next few days. Once the rash appears, it will be around for the next two to three weeks.

The itching and weeping of poison plant rashes can be helped with simple herbal remedies. The Native Americans traditionally used poultices made from the thick, juicy stems of jewelweed (also called wild impatiens or touch-me-not). This can be very effective. In fact, studies show that it works as well as nonprescription hydrocortisone ointment. Herbs that contain tannin have traditionally been recommended because their astringent effect can help relieve itching and dry up oozing blisters. Applying nondistilled witch hazel extract to the affected area is often very helpful. You could also try compresses or poultices made from black tea, bayberry, wood betony, goldenseal, oak bark, mullein, raspberry leaves, yellow dock, or walnut leaves. Some people find that fresh aloe vera gel has a soothing effect.

The itchiness of poison ivy can be soothed by an oatmeal bath. You can purchase colloidal oatmeal (Aveeno brand) at the drugstore, or make it yourself by grinding ordinary rolled oats in a food processor until they are a fine powder. Put 2 cups into a tub of lukewarm water and soak for twenty minutes or so.

If your poison plant rash covers more than 15 percent of your body, if it affects your eyes, mouth, or genitals, if it is very severe, or if it seems infected, see your doctor.

❖ Pregnancy

An unborn baby is most susceptible to harm two to eight weeks after conception, but most women don't know they're pregnant until three or more weeks after conception. That means that if you're pregnant or think you might be, or if you're planning to get pregnant, you need to be very careful about what you consume, starting immediately.

The United States Public Health Service now advises all women capable of becoming pregnant to consume 0.4 milligrams (400 micrograms) of folic acid daily, either from dietary sources or supplements. Folic acid, also called folacin or folate, is one of the B vitamins. Conclusive evidence now shows that folacin helps prevent neural tube defects in unborn children. Because these defects, which can cause spina bifida, anencephaly, and other crippling problems, develop in the first two weeks after conception, it's vital for women to get enough folic acid *before* they become pregnant. Folic acid is found in many healthy foods such as dark green leafy vegetables. Popular food supplements that contain folic acid include brewer's yeast and wheat germ. Even if you regularly eat a good, healthy diet, discuss taking folic acid supplements with your doctor if you are planning to get pregnant. Folic acid needs vitamin B_{12}, niacin, and vitamin C to be used properly by your body, so you might also want to consider adding a daily multivitamin supplement, especially if you are a vegetarian. Don't take megadoses of vitamin or minerals. These can lead to birth defects.

Women who drink alcohol during pregnancy—even as little as one drink a day—can damage their unborn baby. Fetal alcohol syndrome can lead to mental retardation, poor growth, physical defects, and other problems for your child. If you're planning to become pregnant or already are, avoid alcohol. You should also avoid drugs of any sort, if possible. Recreational drugs such as cocaine and marijuana can cause miscarriage, premature birth, and birth defects. Smoking cigarettes during pregnancy can cause you to miscarry or have a low birth weight or premature baby. If you smoke, stop—for your own sake and for your baby's.

Recent studies have found that caffeine in moderation is safe for pregnant women. You can consume up to 300 milligrams a day—that's the equivalent of three 8-ounce cups of coffee, seven 8-ounce cups of tea, or five 12-ounce cans of cola. Many pregnant women switch to mild herbal teas that have no caffeine. Raspberry leaf tea is often recommended as a safe and enjoyable herbal drink during pregnancy. It's high in tannin, however, so to be on the safe side, don't drink more than 3 cups a day. If you want to try raspberry leaf tea, be sure to purchase exactly that at the health food store. Don't mistakenly purchase raspberry-flavored black tea.

Some nonprescription drugs, even aspirin, can cause fetal problems, especially in the first three months of pregnancy. Some women believe that herbal or natural products are harmless alternatives to nonprescription or prescription drugs during pregnancy. Nothing could be farther from the truth. Avoid diuretic herbs such as parsley and goldenrod; avoid any sort of colon cleansing or laxative herbs such as senna, aloe, rhubarb, buckthorn, or cascara sagrada. Many other herbs contain toxic substances that could cause problems such as uterine contractions. Avoid yarrow, sage, wood betony, thyme oil, fenugreek, vervain, chamomile oil, lady's mantle, celery seeds, celery oil, angelica, wormwood, fennel, fennel seeds, goldenseal, lavender, rue, pennyroyal oil, turmeric, juniper, motherwort, basil oil, pokeroot, ginseng, mugwort, myrrh, shepherd's purse, and cinnamon oil. If you wish to use any sort of herbal remedy, discuss it with your doctor first.

Wild yam root, also sometimes called Mexican wild yam, is sometimes recommended by natural medicine practitioners during pregnancy and labor. This is very dangerous. Do not use wild yam root for anything.

Some fluid retention, or edema, is common and normal in pregnancy. But edema can also be a symptom of a serious condition called toxemia, so tell you doctor at once if your hands, legs, feet, or face become swollen or puffy. You can help relieve the discomfort of mild fluid retention by cutting back on salt and resting with your legs elevated. Do not attempt to treat edema or toxemia yourself by taking diuretics or supplements of the amino acid L-methionine.

See also Breast-Feeding; Morning Sickness.

❖ Premenstrual Syndrome (PMS)

Premenstrual syndrome, better known as PMS, refers to a variety of symptoms that women may experience one or two weeks before the start of their menstrual periods. Somewhat less than half of all women have PMS to some degree. For most, the symptoms are minor inconveniences and can be dealt with easily. For about 10 percent of PMS sufferers, however, the symptoms can be a real problem, interfering with family relationships and work. Over 150 PMS symptoms have been identified, but most fall into four groups.

- Nervous tension, irritability, anxiety, mood swings
- Weight gain, swellings of hands or feet, breast tenderness, abdominal bloating
- Headache, craving for sweets, increased appetite, pounding heart, fatigue, dizziness, fainting
- Depression, forgetfulness, crying, confusion, insomnia

PMS symptoms occur before a woman's period begins and they generally improve once menstruation has started. PMS symptoms should not be confused with menstrual cramps and other problems—PMS has a different cause and treatment.

The exact causes of PMS are still unknown, but some research suggests that diet plays a role. Some women find that increasing their intake of vitamin B$_6$ and magnesium can help relieve their symptoms, although why this sometimes helps is still not understood. Popular herbs and food supplements that are high in vitamin B$_6$ include brewer's yeast, wheat germ, alfalfa, bee pollen, dandelion leaves, burdock root, kelp, and red clover flowers. Magnesium is found in alfalfa, chamomile flowers, garlic, red clover flowers, dandelion leaves, bee pollen, and wheat bran. If you wish to try taking supplements of vitamin B$_6$, magnesium, and other vitamins and minerals, discuss them with your doctor first.

Fluid retention is one of the more common and annoying PMS symptoms. Try limiting your salt intake in the days before your period. Mild diuretic herbs, usually taken as teas, can provide some relief by causing increased urination. Dandelion root, parsley, lovage, corn silk, black cohosh, wood betony, goldenrod, and bearberry (uva ursi) are often recommended. Buchu tea, made from the dried leaves of a South African shrub, is popular in Europe as a diuretic; it is also said to be helpful for relieving breast tenderness. Do not use herbal diuretics for more than a few days, and don't use them if you have any sort of chronic medical condition, such as diabetes or high blood pressure. Commercial PMS teas, made from blends of various diuretics and calming herbs, are sold in health food stores. Some women find that a particular brand works well for them.

Evening primrose oil is sometimes recommended for PMS symptoms. This may help some women, particularly those who get sore breasts, but there is little data to support the claim. Raspberry leaf tea is a traditional remedy for PMS and menstrual discomfort. In traditional Chinese medicine, dong quai is recommended. Old European herbals suggest St. John's wort and skullcap.

Cutting back on caffeine could relieve tension, insomnia, and breast tenderness. Avoid alcohol, since it has depressant effects. If you smoke, stop.

❖ Prostate Disease

Roughly the size and shape of a walnut, the prostate is an important gland in the male reproductive system. It is located in front of the rectum and just below the bladder, where it wraps around the urethra, the tube that carries urine from the bladder out through the penis. After a man reaches age forty, and especially after the age of sixty, the prostate may become a source of problems.

Benign prostatic hyperplasia (BPH), or enlarged prostate, eventually develops in about 80 percent of all men. The prostate gland enlarges and squeezes the urethra; this can sometimes cause difficulty in urinating or other urinary tract problems. Enlarged prostate is not a symptom of cancer and it does not lead to cancer.

An herb that has shown some promise for the treatment of benign prostatic hyperplasia is saw palmetto, also called sabal (or by its scientific names *Serenoa serrulata* or *Serenoa repens*). Over-the-counter preparations containing an extract of saw palmetto are used to treat mild BPH symptoms in Canada and Germany. In the United States, however, the Food and Drug Administration does not allow nonprescription remedies containing saw palmetto to be sold as treatments for BPH. It is possible to purchase saw palmetto in the U.S., but any homemade use of it is unlikely to be effective because the active ingredient is not water-soluble. Another plant that is sometimes recommended by herbalists is leaves from an African shrub called *Pygeum africanum*. Only anecdotal evidence suggests that this works, so avoid it. In traditional Chinese medicine, ginseng is recommended for prostate problems.

Some men have found that adding zinc to their diet helps relieve BPH symptoms. Good sources of zinc include wheat germ, kelp, red clover flowers, rose hips, watercress, alfalfa, dandelion leaves, garlic, and burdock root. Discuss adding zinc to your diet, through food or supplements, with your doctor before trying it.

If you have BPH, it is important to drink plenty of fluids and empty your bladder fully when your urinate. This will help prevent bladder infections. Sometimes herbalists recommend mild herbal diuretics such as buchu tea, horsetail, corn silk, and goldenrod for men with BPH. Do not use diuretics to relieve BPH symptoms—drink more fluids instead. If you pass any blood in your urine or develop a urinary tract infection, see your doctor.

The amino acids L-glycine and L-glutamine are sometimes said to help relieve the symptoms of prostate problems. There is no evidence that they do so, and taking supplements of single amino acids could be dangerous to your health.

Prostate cancer is the most common major cancer in American men. Prostate cancer occurs in one out of ten men, but it has no symptoms in its early stages and can usually be cured if it is detected at that point. If you are a male over age forty, it's important to see your doctor for regular checkups.

❖ Psoriasis

Psoriasis, a persistent skin disease that affects millions of people, causes inflammation, scaling, and itchiness. Psoriasis usually begins with little red bumps on the skin. These gradually grow larger and scales form. The top scales flake off easily, but the scales below cause red, itchy patches on the skin. The elbows, knees, groin and genitals, arms, legs, scalp, and nails are the areas most commonly affected. The cause of psoriasis is unknown.

Herbal remedies are sometimes suggested for psoriasis. Angelica, for example, contains psoralens, substances that are used to help some very severe cases of psoriasis. However, eating angelica or applying it to the affected area won't help and is potentially very dangerous. Burdock root is also said to help psoriasis, but there is little evidence that this is so. Dried burdock root has virtually no active ingredients, while the fresh roots and leaves contain little of value. Furthermore, there is no evidence that drinking teas or taking capsules made from red clover flowers, milk thistle, dandelion, or yellow dock have any effect on psoriasis.

Herbal creams or ointments for psoriasis may provide some temporary relief of itching. Tea tree oil is said to be effective for many people; calendula and comfrey ointments are often suggested by herbalists.

Fish oil (EPA) and evening primrose oil (GLA) in very large amounts have helped reduce itching and inflammation for some psoriasis patients. Discuss taking these supplements with your doctor before trying them.

For temporary relief of itching, try a soothing colloidal oatmeal bath. You can purchase colloidal oatmeal (Aveeno brand) at the drugstore, or make it yourself by grinding ordinary rolled oats in a food processor until they are a fine powder. Put 2 cups into a tub of lukewarm water and soak for twenty minutes or so.

❖ Radiation Therapy

Half of all cancer patients are treated with radiation, either alone or in combination with surgery and chemotherapy. In fact, for many cancer patients, radiation therapy is the only treatment needed. Radiation therapy often has unpleasant side effects, mostly because the radiation kills fast-growing cancer cells, which unfortunately also means it affects fast-growing normal cells, especially those in your digestive system. Loss of appetite, difficulty chewing and swallowing, sore throat, nausea, diarrhea, and skin irritation are some of the most common side effects.

Fortunately, modern drugs can help relieve many of the side effects. Anti-emetic drugs, for example, can relieve nausea and vomiting very effectively. Since good nutrition is a must for radiation therapy patients, discuss these drugs with your doctor before beginning therapy. For mild nausea, traditional herbal remedies such as hot peppermint tea or chamomile tea may help. Other herbal remedies for nausea and vomiting could interfere with your treatment, so discuss them with your doctor before you try them.

Patients getting radiation therapy do better and recover faster if they eat well during the treatment period. To cope with a general loss of appetite, eat when you are hungry—whenever that may be. Try having several small meals a day instead of three larger ones. Keep nutritious snacks on hand to nibble on if you feel hungry but don't want much. Choose foods that taste good to you and that are easy to eat. You can liven up bland foods by adding flavorful herbs such as oregano or thyme, but if spicy foods worsen your nausea, avoid hot peppers and other sharp flavorings. If you can eat only a small amount at one time, make sure you get the maximum number of calories you can from the meal. Try adding cream or milk to canned cream soups instead of water. Eggnog, milk shakes, or prepared liquid supplements are tasty, nutritious, and easy to swallow. Cream sauce, butter, or melted cheese on your vegetables will add calories and flavor. If you can't handle solid foods, drink plenty of nutritious liquids. Try adding powdered nonfat milk, plain yogurt, honey, or prepared liquid supplements to your drinks. Some patients like to add a big spoonful of wheat germ.

If you are having radiation to the head or neck area, you may have redness and irritation in the mouth, dry mouth, difficulty in swallowing, changes in taste, or nausea. Avoid spices and coarse foods, such as raw vegetables, dry crackers, and nuts. Don't drink alcohol, and avoid sugary foods. If your mouth is dry, sip cool water throughout the day; some patients find that carbonated beverages help relieve dry mouth better than plain water. Avoid tea and herbal teas that contain tannin, such as raspberry leaf tea. Sucking on sugar-free candy or chewing sugar-free gum may also help. Moisten foods with sauces or gravy to make eating easier. It's very important to take proper care of your teeth during this time. Your doctor will work with you and your dentist to help you with dental care. Do not substitute herbal mouthwashes or natural toothpastes for the products your dentist prescribes. Discuss the use of herbal remedies for mouth sores with your doctor or dentist before you try them.

Radiation therapy in the chest area can make swallowing difficult or painful. Try mashing or pureeing your foods or adding gravies or sauces to make them softer. Avoid spicy foods and foods that are dry and rough, such as crackers or nuts. Cut your food into small, bite-sized pieces. Discuss liquid food supplements with your doctor if solid food is too uncomfortable to eat.

Nausea, vomiting, and diarrhea can be serious problems during radiation therapy to the stomach and abdomen. If you feel nauseous after a treatment, try not eating for several hours before the next treatment. Some patients handle the radiation better on an empty stomach. After your treatment, you may find it helpful to wait one or two hours before eating again. If your doctor or dietitian prescribes a special diet, try to stick to it. To deal with nausea, eat six or more small meals or snacks throughout the day rather than three larger ones. Avoid foods that are fried, fatty, or have a strong smell. Drink plenty of cool liquids such as plain water, diluted fruit juices, and mild herbal teas between meals. After three or four weeks of radiation therapy, you may develop diarrhea. To deal with this, your doctor may prescribe medication and some changes in your diet. Try a clear liquid diet as soon as the diarrhea starts or you feel it might start. Drink plenty of clear fluids such as water, apple juice, diluted fruit nectars, and weak tea (mild herbal teas such as peppermint and chamomile are good); plain gelatin and clear broths are also helpful. Avoid milk and milk products, coffee, and alcohol. When the diarrhea begins to subside, try eating small amounts of low-fiber foods such as bananas, cottage cheese, rice, applesauce, mashed potatoes, and dry toast. Try to eat foods that are high in potassium, such as bananas, wheat germ, blackstrap molasses, brewer's yeast, garlic, orange juice, and apricots, since you may lose a lot of this mineral from diarrhea. Alfalfa juice, bee pollen, chamomile flowers, and kelp also have potassium. If you would like to try any herbal remedies for diarrhea, discuss them with your doctor first.

The skin over the area receiving radiation therapy may become irritated, very dry, red, or feel burned. If this happens, be sure to tell your doctor. He or she will probably prescribe a special ointment to help the problem. Use *only* this ointment. Do not apply any other cream or ointment to the area.

Herbalists sometimes suggest that radiation therapy patients take daily doses of the antibiotic herb echinacea. This is said to help the patient tolerate the radiation better and to help prevent secondary infections. Kelp, alfalfa, and chaparral are also said to help radiation therapy patients. There is no evidence that any of these herbs have value for this purpose, and chaparral is not considered safe by the Food and Drug Administration. If you want to try echinacea or any other herbal remedy during radiation therapy, discuss it with your doctor first.

Some medications, including over-the-counter drugs such as cold pills, can interfere with the beneficial effects of radiation therapy. So can many herbal remedies or large doses of vitamin and mineral supplements, so be sure to consult your doctor before taking any drugs, herbs, or supplements.

Fortunately, the side effects of radiation therapy begin to go away once the therapy stops. For most people, radiation therapy is given five days a week for six or seven weeks. It may take some time after that for your appetite and strength to return fully.

See also Chemotherapy.

❖ Raynaud's Disease

If you have Raynaud's disease, the small arteries that supply blood to your hands and sometimes your feet become supersensitive to cold. These small blood vessels suddenly contract when exposed to cold air. This reduces the flow of blood to your extremities and makes your fingers and toes become pale or bluish and numb. They change back to their normal color and regain feeling when you warm up. Raynaud's disease is quite common. It usually affects women, starting in early adulthood. Although it is sometimes caused by an underlying problem, such as scleroderma or working with heavy power tools, most often there is no known cause. Over the course of many years, Raynaud's disease can lead to weakened fingers and a diminished sense of touch, but generally it is more of an annoyance than a serious problem.

The best way to relieve the symptoms of Raynaud's disease is to dress appropriately in cold weather. Another good self-help step is to stop smoking. Hot foods and drinks can help keep you warm in cold weather, with the exception of coffee, tea, and other beverages with caffeine—the caffeine can constrict your blood vessels. Spicy foods made with cayenne or chili peppers can also help warm you up. Garlic and onions may help relieve your symptoms, since these foods can help improve your circulation.

Avoid alcoholic beverages. The alcohol temporarily opens the blood vessels in your hands and feet and may make you feel warmer for a few minutes, but after a short time the alcohol causes your core body temperature to drop, leading to a further reduction in blood flow to your extremities.

Because omega-3 fatty acids (fish oil) can improve circulation, you might try adding more deep sea fish such as tuna, mackerel, and herring to your diet, or try a daily fish-oil capsule. Don't take fish oil capsules if you're diabetic.

The herbs butcher's broom, ginkgo biloba, and pau d'arco are all said to help improve blood flow, which could help the symptoms of Raynaud's disease. Butcher's broom has become popular in Europe, and capsules are now available in American health food stores, but its therapeutic effects, if any, have not been proven. Ginkgo biloba extract is another popular European remedy said to be helpful to the circulatory system, particularly for the elderly. Some evidence suggests this is true, so it is possible that using the extract, in liquid, capsule, or tablet form, could help relieve Raynaud's disease symptoms. Use caution: Very large doses could cause nausea, diarrhea, and other side effects. Don't take ginkgo biloba if you are taking any sort of blood-thinning medication. Pau d'arco bark, an herb from South America, is ineffective and possibly dangerous—avoid it.

❖ Shingles

Like chicken pox, shingles, an unpleasant ailment characterized by pain and skin blisters, is caused by the herpes zoster virus. Once you've had chicken pox, the virus can remain dormant in certain nerve cells in you body. Later in life, the virus can reactivate (especially if your immune system is depressed) and cause shingles. The disease afflicts about 20 percent of the population at some point and is more likely to occur in people over age fifty.

The first symptom is usually a burning pain or tingling and extreme sensitivity in one area of the skin. After a few days, a red rash erupts that soon turns into blisters that resemble chicken pox. The blisters usually last for two or three weeks, then crust over and begin to disappear, but the severe pain that goes with them may last longer.

The blisters of shingles most commonly appear on the trunk and buttocks. If blisters appear on the face or nose, they could involve the eye region and cause permanent eye damage. If you have shingles and develop blisters on the face, see an eye doctor at once.

Older people who have had shingles sometimes develop postherpetic neuralgia, a complication where the pain of shingles continues long after the blisters have gone away. Over-the-counter ointments containing capsicum, better known as cayenne pepper, often relieve the pain when applied to the affected area, although it can take a few days of regular application for the ointment to be effective. Never use capsicum ointment on or near the eyes or mucous membranes.

Although shingles is far less contagious than chicken pox, someone who has shingles may transmit chicken pox to someone who has never had it. If you have shingles, avoid contact with very young children, pregnant women, and people whose immune systems are depressed, such as cancer or AIDS patients.

Most people who have shingles get better in a few weeks without medication, although your doctor may prescribe the antiviral drug acyclovir. To treat the symptoms, doctors recommend painkillers such as ibuprofen, and calamine lotion, cold compresses, and soothing baths in colloidal oatmeal. You can purchase colloidal oatmeal (Aveeno brand) at the drugstore, or make it yourself by grinding ordinary rolled oats in a food processor until they are a fine powder. Put 2 cups in to a tub of lukewarm water and soak for twenty minutes or so.

The herpes zoster virus is related to the herpes virus that causes cold sores and genital herpes. It is possible that eating foods containing the amino acid arginine, including many seeds, nuts, and grains, could worsen your shingles symptoms. The amino acid lysine seems to inhibit the herpes virus. Some shingles sufferers find that supplemental lysine, available in capsules at health food stores, helps relieve their symptoms. Try 500 milligrams a day until the symptoms go away.

See also Cold Sores; Herpes.

❖ Sinusitis

Your sinuses—cavities in the cheek bones found around and behind your nose—are lined with mucus membranes, just as the inside of your nostrils are. If the sinus membranes become inflamed, they swell up and close off the narrow passages that connect the sinuses to the nasal cavity. Sinusitis occurs when infected material builds up inside the sinus cavities, causing the most common sinusitis symptom, a severe headache. Other symptoms of sinusitis include coughing, tiredness, stuffy nose, bad breath, bad-tasting post-nasal drip, and thick, colored mucus.

Many people get occasional sinusitis, often after having a cold. It usually goes away by itself after a week or so. Some people develop chronic sinusitis as a result of allergies or a structural abnormality of the sinuses. If you have severe or frequent sinusitis, see your doctor. Antibiotics, decongestants, or painkillers may help relieve the symptoms.

Some easy self-help steps can also be taken to help relieve sinusitis discomfort. Try a daily dose of echinacea to help fight the infection. Inhaling steam scented with eucalyptus, thyme, or lavender oil often helps relieve congestion and eases sinus headaches.

Drink plenty of liquids—six to eight glasses every day. This helps thin the mucus and makes it easier to expel. Hot liquids in general help improve mucus flow, thus relieving congestion. Hot herbal teas, such a peppermint, chamomile, rose hips, goldenseal, raspberry leaves, and red clover flowers are all good choices. Chicken soup contains the amino acid cysteine, which helps thin mucus. Tea made from ma huang, also known as ephedra, is a popular Chinese herbal remedy that helps relieve congestion. Avoid ma huang if you have high blood pressure, heart disease, glaucoma, or are taking an MAO-inhibiting (antidepressant) drug. Eating spicy foods containing lots of garlic, cayenne pepper, or horseradish can help relieve your symptoms, since these flavorings act as natural decongestants. Eating foods made with lots of fresh ginger is an effective approach recommended by traditional Chinese herbal medicine.

If you smoke, stop. Cigarette smoke is very irritating to the sinuses. Avoid alcohol as well. It can make the symptoms worse and could also interact badly with any other medicines you are taking.

See also Allergies; Hay Fever.

❖ Smoking

Cigarette smoking is directly responsible for the deaths of 400,000 Americans every year, and indirectly responsible for more deaths and illness. Cigarette smoking causes lung cancer, heart disease, emphysema, chronic bronchitis, and a number of other fatal illnesses. If you smoke, at some point you are certain to have health problems caused by your habit.

Smokers know they should quit, but they smoke anyway. One reason is that the nicotine in tobacco smoke is an addictive drug, and addictions are hard to break. If you are truly motivated to quit, however, you can. Here are some hints from the American Lung Association:

- Set a target date for quitting.
- Keep a smoking diary. If you know when and why you smoke, you can change your habits more easily.
- Smoke fewer cigarettes each day as you approach your target date.
- Postpone the urge for a cigarette. If you wait even five minutes after the urge strikes, it will probably pass without your lighting up.
- Chew sugarless gum instead of smoking.
- Buy only one pack of cigarettes at a time.

Several herbal remedies are sometimes suggested to help people stop smoking. Lobelia, an herb that has some effects that are similar to the nicotine in tobacco, is found in some over-the-counter products. Sold as tablets, lozenges, or chewing gum, these products claim to ease tobacco withdrawal symptoms, making it easier to quit smoking—but there is little evidence to substantiate this.

Ginseng, as a tea or capsules, is recommended by traditional Chinese herbalists. European herbalists recommend valerian tea for its sedative effect. In Native American herbal lore, calamus root is recommended for a variety of stomach ailments; modern herbalists sometimes recommend it for people who want to stop smoking. Calamus root (also known as sweet flag) is a known carcinogen, however, and its use as a food or food additive is banned by the Food and Drug Administration. Don't use it.

Some ex-smokers swear that drinking a lot of citrus juice for a couple of weeks after they quit helped them get through that difficult time. Taking 1,000 milligrams a day of vitamin C seems to have a similar effect.

Doctors know a great deal about the damaging effects of tobacco smoke. Other types of smoke can be equally, if not more, dangerous. Clove or other herbal cigarettes are as bad for you as tobacco. Don't smoke anything.

❖ Sore Throat

A scratchy, painful sore throat is a common symptom with a variety of possible causes. It often accompanies a cold, the flu, or hay fever. A sore throat can also be caused by smoking too much or breathing smoky or polluted air. A sore throat along with fever, headache, pain when you swallow, and sore glands in your jaw and throat might indicate tonsillitis, strep throat, or mononucleosis. If you suspect your sore throat is caused by one of these illnesses, see your doctor.

In general, drinking a lot of liquids will help ease your sore throat by keeping the tissues moist. Mild herbal teas, water, and nonacidic fruit juices are all good choices. Favorite herbal teas for sore throats include chamomile, goldenseal, sage, and raspberry leaf. Horehound lozenges and syrups have a soothing effect, as do slippery elm bark and marshmallow. Avoid coltsfoot tea. This may contain dangerous carcinogens.

Many people find that lukewarm beverages are best, but cold or hot drinks may feel better to you. Honey, lemon, and tea (plain or herbal) make a soothing combination. For a more potent mixture, try substituting fresh grated horseradish for the lemon.

Old-fashioned gargling can help a sore throat. Try gargling with 8 ounces of warm water and 1 teaspoon salt or lemon juice. Don't swallow this. Repeat several times a day. A gargle often recommended by herbalists is 10 drops of echinacea tincture in 8 ounces of warm water. Repeat twice a day, swallowing the mixture each time. You could also try gargling several times a day with weak sage tea, which can be swallowed if you wish.

See also Colds.

❖ Sties

A sty forms when the root of one of your eyelashes becomes infected. The sty, a red, pus-filled swelling on your eyelid, can be quite painful and unsightly. In most cases, you can deal with a sty yourself. As soon as you notice it, apply hot compresses to the sty frequently to help bring it to a head. Plain water works well, but you could also try soaking the compress in herbal teas such as goldenseal, calendula, or raspberry leaves. When you notice a white head of pus on the swelling, use clean tweezers to pull out the eyelash. This will release the pus and relieve the swelling. Never squeeze the sty. Wash the eyelid thoroughly with soap and water; clean the tweezers as well.

If you get sties often, or if more than one eyelash is involved, see your doctor.

See also Eye Problems.

❖ Stomach Cancer

While the incidence of lung cancer has been rising sharply, the incidence of stomach cancer in the United States has dropped sharply over the past fifty years. Due to modern refrigeration and freezing, most people now eat far fewer foods that have been smoked, preserved in salt, or pickled. These foods have been directly linked to stomach cancer.

Some herbs may have a preventive effect against stomach cancer. Studies in Japan have shown that people who drink a lot of tea have a lower incidence of stomach cancer than those who drink less. The effect is most pronounced if you drink a lot of green (Chinese) tea, although black tea is also helpful. One reason is probably the high vitamin C content of green tea.

Other studies in Japan have shown that a daily bowl of miso soup, made from soybean paste, could cut the risk of stomach cancer by more than half. Onions and garlic could also reduce your risk. Studies in China, where stomach cancer is common, have shown that a daily serving of scallions, onion, garlic, or chives reduces the risk of stomach cancer by nearly half.

❖ Stress

Life is full of mildly stressful situations that most people can deal with routinely. Occasionally, people must cope with situations that cause more severe stress: major illness, family difficulties, financial worries, and the like. When you are under severe stress, your body responds with physical changes. Your blood pressure and heart rate go up; you may have headaches, back pain, digestive problems, or feel tired all the time. On the emotional level, you could have insomnia, feel anxious, and be unable to relax. In general, being under stress for long periods of time can weaken your immune system and make you more vulnerable to illness. Stress can also worsen some chronic problems such as asthma, eczema, and psoriasis.

Stress is a major factor in modern life. The vague, uncomfortable physical symptoms it produces send many people to the doctor and make diazepam (Valium) one of the most prescribed drugs in the country. If you are experiencing major stress symptoms, and you and your doctor have ruled out any medical cause, some simple self-help techniques and herbal remedies could help. Getting regular exercise can make a big difference. Even a short daily walk of just twenty minutes or so can help you relax and get a better perspective on your worries. Making time for yourself can also help. Try to set aside an hour a day for exercise and relaxation, even if it means cutting back on some other activity. Another important way to reduce stress is to get enough sleep. If you are so busy that you can't get eight hours of sleep a night, it might be time to reconsider your schedule. Sacrificing sleep and feeling tired all the time will make you feel more stressed.

A good, nutritious diet and a regular meal schedule can also help alleviate stress. Try cutting back on caffeine and alcohol—you'll sleep better. If you smoke, stop.

Many herbs, usually in the form of hot teas, are recommended to help you relax. Valerian, which has a sedative effect, can be helpful at bedtime, but should be avoided when you need to be alert. Other soothing herbs include catnip, chamomile, peppermint, raspberry leaves, lavender, rose hips, lemon balm, and vervain. St. John's wort oil may help relieve anxiety. In traditional Chinese herbal medicine, ginseng is often suggested for stress. It is a mild stimulant, so avoid it before bedtime.

See also Anxiety; Depression; Insomnia; Premenstrual Syndrome (PMS).

❖ Stroke and Stroke Prevention

A stroke occurs when one of the blood vessels to the brain bursts or become clogged. The rupture or blockage keeps the brain from getting the blood flow it needs. As a result, the affected area starts to die. The effects can include severe losses in mental and bodily functions and even death.

Stroke is now the third largest cause of death in America, but stroke deaths have been dropping in recent years. The two main reasons for this are improved medical care for stroke victims and better treatment of high blood pressure.

The warning signals of stroke are easy to detect. If you notice any of the symptoms below, get medical attention at once:

- Sudden weakness, numbness, or paralysis of the face, arm, and leg, especially on one side of the body
- Sudden dimness or loss of vision, particularly in one eye
- Loss of speech or trouble talking or understanding speech
- Dizziness, unsteadiness, or sudden falls, especially along with any of the above symptoms

A stroke is a medical emergency. Call 911 for help at once if you suspect a stroke. Stroke-related brain damage gets worse the longer the stroke goes untreated.

About 10 percent of all strokes are preceded by a warning sign called a transient ischemic attack (TIA) days or even weeks before a major stroke. TIAs occur when a blood clot temporarily blocks an artery and cuts off the blood supply to the brain for a short time. TIAs usually last from a few minutes to a few hours. The symptoms are the same as for stroke, but they generally go away within twenty-four hours.

If you experience a TIA, you are likely to have a stroke soon. See your doctor at once.

Some of the risk factors for stroke are beyond control. Simply getting older, being a man, and being African-American mean that you are more likely to have a stroke. People with diabetes are also more likely to have strokes, so it's important to keep your diabetes under control. If you've already had a stroke, you are more likely to have another one, and if you have high blood pressure and fail to control the problem, you are a good candidate for a stroke. If your blood cholesterol is too high or if you are obese, your chances of a stroke are high. If you smoke, stop. If you have more than two alcoholic drinks a day, cut back. Light or moderate drinking may reduce your stroke risk, but heavy drinking definitely increases it.

An extract made from the leaves of the ginkgo biloba tree is widely used in Europe for diseases that affect the flow of blood to the brain. Careful study has shown that large doses of ginkgo biloba are effective for improving blood flow and for reducing clotting time, particularly for elderly patients. It is possible that daily doses of ginkgo biloba could help prevent strokes. Doses large enough to be useful can often produce side effects such as diarrhea, nausea, and vomiting. If this occurs, reduce the dosage or stop taking ginkgo biloba. If you already take any sort of blood-thinning drug (including low doses of aspirin), talk to your doctor before trying ginkgo biloba. Although ginkgo biloba is available by prescription and over the counter in Germany, it is not approved as a drug in the United States. It is sold in health food stores as a food or food supplement, however.

It's possible that green (Chinese) tea may have a preventative effect against stroke. Studies in Japan have shown that women who drink a lot of green tea have a lower incidence of stroke than those who drink less of it. Green tea has a lot of vitamin C and other antioxidant substances, which could be what makes it effective.

Omega-3 fatty acids (fish oil) could be another way to reduce your stroke risk. Fish oil may help thin your blood, which reduces the chance of a blood clot blocking the flow to your brain. The best dietary source of omega-3 fatty acids is deep sea fish such as tuna, mackeral, and herring; you could also try supplemental capsules.

Onions, garlic, and scallions all contain blood-thinning substances that could help prevent the blood clots that lead to strokes. If you are at risk for stroke, try adding onions and garlic to your diet or consider taking garlic capsules.

See also Diabetes; High Blood Pressure; High Cholesterol; Obesity.

❖ Sunburn

Excessive exposure to the sun's ultraviolet rays causes sunburn—skin that is reddened, swollen, or even blistered. At best, sunburn is a painful nuisance; however, a serious sunburn can be extremely uncomfortable and even dangerous. Excess exposure to the sun can also lead to skin cancer later in life.

Cold compresses are helpful for relieving the discomfort of sunburn. A soft cloth dipped in plain cold water and placed on the affected area can be very soothing. Replace the cloth with a fresh one every few minutes, and continue the treatment for ten to fifteen minutes at a time, several times a day. You could try replacing the plain cold water with strong, cold tea. For minor sunburn, try applying lavender oil, distilled witch hazel, aloe vera gel, or St. John's wort oil to the area. Calendula cream can also be very soothing.

If your sunburn covers a large area, try a cool bath in plain water. Adding a cup of white vinegar or a generous handful of baking soda to the bathwater may give you additional relief. Colloidal oatmeal in the bath can be very soothing. Purchase Aveeno brand colloidal oatmeal at the drugstore or make your own by grinding ordinary rolled oats in a food processor until they are a fine powder. Put 1 cup into a tub of cool water and soak for twenty minutes or so.

The discomfort of your sunburn should be a reminder to protect yourself from the sun. To avoid burning, use a sunscreen with an SPF (sun protection factor) of 15. Remember that you can get a sunburn even on cloudy days and in the winter, too. Wear sunscreen if you are active outdoors when there is snow or ice on the ground.

❖ Swimmer's Ear

Swimming is one of the best exercises you can do, especially if you have arthritis. Swimming places little strain on the joints, so you have a low chance of injury. Frequent swimmers (or people who swim in dirty water) do often develop one minor ailment, however: swimmer's ear (otitis externa). Frequent excessive moisture in the ear canal can make the outer ear more susceptible to infection. The usual symptoms are itching and redness in the ear canal, followed later by pain and, sometimes, a discharge of pus. If you have an outer ear infection, see your doctor. He or she will probably prescribe antibiotics (or possibly an antifungal) to clear it up. While you have the infection, it's important to keep your ears dry. Avoid swimming and use ear plugs when bathing.

Once the infection is gone, you can resume swimming, but wear a swim cap or ear plugs to prevent reinfection. (If your infection was from swimming in dirty or polluted water, find somewhere else to swim.) Another way to prevent a recurrence of swimmer's ear is a remedy known to the ancient Egyptians. After you swim, dry your outer ear thoroughly and, using a clean dropper, place a few drops of distilled white vinegar into each ear.

See also Ear Infections.

❖ Thyroid Problems

Your thyroid is a butterfly-shaped gland found at the base of your throat. The thyroid produces a hormone called thyroxine, which affects the rate at which chemical reactions occur in your body. If your thyroid produces too much thyroxine, you develop hyperthyroidism; if it produces too little, you develop hypothyroidism.

Hyperthyroidism is fairly uncommon, but occurs more frequently in women than men. The usual symptoms include agitation, insomnia, weight loss, sensitivity to heat, diarrhea, and possibly goiter, or swelling of the thyroid gland. Sometimes herbalists recommend treatment with bugle weed, but this is poor advice. See your doctor if you suspect hyperthyroidism.

Hypothyroidism (also sometimes called myxedema) develops slowly, often over months or years. The usual symptoms include fatigue, sensitivity to cold, aches and pains, heavy menstrual periods, weight gain, and constipation. Hypothyroidism is not uncommon, although natural medicine practitioners diagnose it much more often than do orthodox physicians. Middle-aged women are the most likely to have the problem.

Herbalists sometimes suggest kelp or other seaweed as a treatment for hypothyroidism. The iodine in the seaweed is said to help stimulate the thyroid. While it is true that a serious iodine deficiency can cause goiter, this deficiency is extremely rare in the United States, where nearly everyone gets ample iodine from iodized table salt (sea salt has very little). Too much iodine can actually inhibit the production of thyroid hormones. Other remedies include the herbs goldenseal and black cohosh and supplements of the amino acid L-tyrosine. However, none of these are likely to be effective. If you have or suspect hypothyroidism, see your doctor. Most people respond very well to hormone replacement medication.

❖ Tinnitus

Tinnitus, an irritating problem that usually affects older adults, is often described as a ringing in the ears, but the sound can also be a buzz, pop, or hum. Prolonged exposure to high noise levels is one cause of tinnitus; people who work around jackhammers, jet engines, heavy machinery, and other noisy apparatus are more likely to develop it. According to the American Tinnitus Association, about fifty million Americans have tinnitus to some degree; of that number, twelve million have it severely enough to seek medical help. Tinnitus does not cause hearing loss, although most people who have hearing loss experience some tinnitus. More than 200 prescription and nonprescription drugs list tinnitus as a potential side effect.

Alcohol, nicotine, caffeine, some prescription drugs, and aspirin can all make tinnitus worse and should be avoided. If you have tinnitus, avoid willow bark, apples, and most berries. These contain natural salicylates, the same substance found in aspirin, and could make your tinnitus worse.

Ginkgo biloba extract, in tablet or liquid form, can be very helpful for people with tinnitus, especially those who are elderly. Ginkgo probably works by dilating the blood vessels and improving blood flow. Large doses are needed, however, and ginkgo could interfere with other medications you might be taking, such as blood thinners. Discuss using ginkgo biloba with your doctor before you try it.

❖ Tooth Care

The most important steps you can take to prevent cavities, gum disease, and other dental ailments are regular brushing and flossing and a visit to your dentist twice a year for a checkup and professional cleaning.

Although a bewildering array of toothpastes is available, dentists agree that any one that has fluoride is fine. This mineral helps strengthen the protective enamel of your teeth throughout your life and is routinely added to drinking water in most communities. The beneficial effects of fluoride can be seen in today's sharply lower cavity rates for young children. Nearly half have no cavities in their permanent teeth. If you choose a natural toothpaste that does not contain fluoride or if you drink only pure bottled water, you will not get any of the protective benefits of added fluoride.

A number of different herbs and other substances have been traditionally recommended for cleaning the teeth. Green (Chinese) tea contains antibiotic substances that help kill the germs responsible for dental decay and gum disease. Bloodroot (also called sanguinaria) is often used in natural mouthwashes and toothpastes; it is an effective treatment for preventing dental plaque. Licorice root contains glycyrrhizin, a compound that may be effective against tooth decay. In India, fresh curry leaves are often rubbed against the teeth as a way to clean them. Neem, another Indian herb, is a common ingredient in natural toothpastes; it has natural antibiotic and antiplaque ingredients. Propolis, a brown, resinous substance made by honeybees, is also sometimes used as an ingredient in natural toothpastes; it is said to have antibiotic properties.

Clove oil can temporarily relieve the discomfort of a toothache. Soak a cotton ball in the oil and rub it directly against the aching tooth and gums. An effective short-term remedy used by Native Americans is chewing the bark of the prickly ash tree. See your dentist as soon as possible if you have a toothache, even a mild one.

See also Bad Breath; Gum Disease.

❖ Ulcers

An ulcer is a craterlike sore on the lining of your digestive tract. Most ulcers occur in the duodenum, the first part of your small intestine, although they can also occur in your stomach or in your esophagus. Are you more likely to get ulcers if you are under a lot of stress? Surprisingly, the answer is no. Hard-driving executive types are no more likely to get ulcers than anyone else. If you smoke, however, you are more likely to get ulcers. Ulcers affect some nineteen million Americans at least once in their lifetime. They most commonly first appear in people between the ages of thirty and fifty.

In many, if not most, cases, ulcers are caused by a bacteria. However, ulcers may also be caused by damage to the membranes that line your digestive tract. Acid and other digestive fluids from your stomach then burn the damaged area and cause a sore. Some anti-inflammatory drugs, such as aspirin, ibuprofen, and prescription drugs for arthritis can damage the stomach lining and cause ulcers.

Ulcer symptoms are fairly easy to recognize because they are so uncomfortable. The most common symptom is a gnawing or burning pain in the abdomen between the lower end of the breastbone and the navel. The pain often occurs between meals and in the early hours of the morning. It may last for a few minutes to a few hours and is often temporarily relieved by eating or taking an antacid. Other ulcer symptoms include nausea, vomiting, and appetite loss.

Doctors used to treat ulcers by prescribing a bland diet and urging patients to drink milk or cream. Unfortunately, this often actually worsened the problem, since the calcium in the milk stimulated the patients to make more stomach acid. Today, the treatment is usually a normal diet combined with antibiotics and drugs that reduce the production of stomach acid; nonprescription liquid antacids are also often recommended.

Drinking alcohol will aggravate an ulcer and keep it from healing as quickly. If you drink alcohol, do so in moderation and never on an empty stomach. Caffeine can also slow down the healing process, so avoid caffeinated coffee, tea, and other beverages. Eating small, frequent meals when you're having ulcer pain may also help. If you have an ulcer caused by a prescription or over-the-counter drug, talk to your doctor about reducing the dosage, taking the drug with meals, taking an over-the-counter antacid liquid, and other possible ways to help deal with the problem.

Some herbal treatments for ulcers can be effective. Licorice root *(Glycyrrhiza glabra)* can be very helpful for peptic (stomach) ulcers. It is usually taken as a tea made from 1 teaspoonful of the licorice root steeped in 1/2 cup of water for five minutes. Strain before drinking; take 1/2 cup three times a day after meals. However, licorice root can cause you to retain fluids. Don't use it if you have high blood pressure, heart disease, liver disease, or diabetes. Stop using licorice root if you notice any swelling in your face, hands, or feet, and don't use it for longer than four weeks. Some patients report that drinking fresh cabbage juice helps their symptoms, although there's not much scientific basis for this. In traditional Chinese medicine, ginger and ginseng are often recommended for ulcers. Ginger is particularly effective for some patients, perhaps because it reduces the production of stomach acid. Gentian and strong chamomile tea are traditional European herbal remedies that can be helpful. Other remedies that are sometimes recommended by herbalists include alfalfa (juice or tablets), red clover flowers, and kelp, but these herbs are unlikely to provide any relief.

See also Heartburn; Indigestion; Nausea.

❖ Urinary Tract Infections

The most common symptom of a urinary tract infection (UTI) is a frequent urge to urinate and a painful, burning sensation during urination. Despite the urge to urinate, you might pass only a small amount of urine, and the urine itself may have a bad odor and appear milky, cloudy, or even have a reddish tinge of blood. Women often have pain or uncomfortable pressure above the pubic bone. An overall feeling of being tired and ill is common. However, children with UTIs often have no symptoms aside from increased urination or have symptoms that are confused with other illnesses.

Women are especially prone to these painful infections. By some estimates, up to 20 percent of all women will have a UTI some time in their lives. Women get them much more often than men because they have a shorter urethra, so bacteria have a shorter distance to travel to enter the bladder. UTIs are unusual in men. When they do occur, they are usually the result of a kidney stone or an enlarged prostate gland. People with diabetes are also more prone to UTIs because the high levels of sugar in their urine are a fertile breeding ground for bacteria.

If you have a urinary tract infection, see your doctor. He or she will probably prescribe antibiotics, which usually clear up the worst symptoms within a day or two. Even after you start feeling better, it's important to finish taking your medicine to avoid recurring infections, and to keep from developing a kidney infection. In addition, there are some self-help steps and herbal remedies you can take to relieve symptoms and help prevent a recurrence.

Many women find that they can relieve the pain of a UTI with a warm bath or heating pad. Drinking lots of fluids helps by flushing bacteria out of the urinary tract, but avoid caffeine (especially coffee) and alcohol, which are irritating. Try to drink six to eight glasses of liquid a day, and make one or two of those glasses cranberry or blueberry juice. Compounds in these juices have been shown to help prevent UTI recurrences by keeping bacteria from sticking to the walls of the bladder.

Uva ursi (also called bearberry) is a traditional herbal treatment for urinary tract infections. The leaves of this plant have an antiseptic and diuretic effect that can be helpful for bladder problems. Because uva ursi also contains large amounts of tannins, which can cause stomach upsets, herbalists usually recommend making a cold infusion from the leaves. For the best results, soak 1/2 cup of uva ursi leaves in 2 quarts of cold water for twelve to twenty-four hours. Strain before using. The usual dose is 1 cup of the tea up to six times a day.

Many of the herbs often suggested for urinary tract infections have diuretic effects—that is, they increase the volume of urine you produce. Diuretic herbs include juniper oil, parsley, lovage, corn silk, goldenrod, and buchu tea. All are mildly effective; buchu tea may also have an antiseptic effect. Juniper should be avoided by pregnant women and people with kidney disease. Gentian root tea is a traditional Chinese herbal treatment for urinary tract problems.

About four out of five women who have a UTI develop another one within eighteen months. To help prevent a recurrence, drink lots of fluids as discussed above. Don't put off urinating when you feel the need, and try to empty your bladder completely each time. Wipe from front to back to prevent bacteria from entering the vagina or urethra. Always urinate shortly before and after sexual intercourse. Avoid using feminine hygiene sprays and scented douches. If you use a diaphragm and get urinary tract infections often, discuss alternative methods of birth control with your doctor.

See also Vaginitis.

❖ Vaginitis

A general term for any inflammation of the vagina, vaginitis is usually caused by a yeast infection (candidiasis) or by a bacterial infection. (See the section on Yeast Infections for more information about candidiasis.) Sometimes vaginitis is caused by an irritant, such as laundry soap or feminine hygiene products.

Vaginitis symptoms can vary, depending upon the type of bacteria. One common kind causes a white, gray, or yellowish vaginal discharge, a fishy odor in the genital area, itching, and a slight redness or swelling of the vagina and vulva. Another common type of bacteria causes a watery, yellowish, greenish bubbly discharge, an unpleasant odor, and pain and itching when urinating. Symptoms are most likely to appear after your menstrual period.

Vaginitis is usually treated with antibiotic pills or an antibiotic cream. Don't insert yogurt into the vagina if you have a bacterial infection. It will make it worse.

Some women find that the symptoms of itchiness are relieved by soaking in a warm bath that has 1 cup of white vinegar added. Diluted tea tree oil applied directly to the itchy area often helps relieve the itchiness. Some traditional herbal remedies that may help vaginal itching include rosewater, lavender oil, and lady's mantle ointment. Goldenseal, taken as a tea, is a traditional herbal treatment for vaginal discharge.

Diabetics are more likely to get vaginitis. Good hygiene and careful attention to your blood sugar levels can help keep the problem under control.

Irritant vaginitis usually causes itching, redness, and a yellowish or white discharge. Common irritants include laundry detergent, fabric softeners, feminine deodorants, douches, bubble baths, colored toilet paper, scented tampons, latex from condoms or diaphragms, spermicides, or physical irritation (from bike riding, for example). Try different brands of laundry products and avoid putting anything scented or colored near your genitals. Most doctors suggest avoiding feminine hygiene products. They're rarely necessary, and they can cause irritation. If your birth control method is the problem, discuss alternative methods with your doctor.

In general, you can reduce the risk of vaginitis and help prevent recurrences by keeping your genital area clean and dry. Wear all-cotton underpants during the day, and skip underpants altogether at night. Avoid wearing tight trousers, leggings, panty hose, bathing suits, leotards, biking shorts, and other tightly fitting apparel for long periods. Whenever possible, wear loose clothing made from natural fabrics. Stay out of hot tubs—the shared warm water is a perfect medium for passing germs around. If you have vaginitis, use a condom when you have intercourse to avoid passing infection to your partner.

See also Herpes; Urinary Tract Infections; Yeast Infections.

❖ Varicose Veins

Twisted, swollen varicose veins in your legs can be very painful. They are often tender to the touch, and the skin at the site of the swollen vein may be itchy. Your whole leg may ache and your feet may become swollen; standing or walking for even a short period may make both legs feel sore and tired. In severe cases, skin ulcers can form over the vein. More worrisome is the possibility of the vein rupturing or of blood clots forming.

In many cases, severe varicose veins can be treated in the doctor's office by sclerotherapy. This involves injecting a solution into the vein that causes the vessel to be absorbed by the body. In some cases, you will need a surgical procedure to remove the vein. In either case, other veins take over the job of circulating the blood.

Some self-help techniques can relieve the discomfort of varicose veins. Most doctors recommend staying off your feet as much as possible, wearing support stockings, and keeping your legs elevated, especially at night. Try raising up the foot of your bed six inches with bricks or wooden blocks. Keep your weight at normal levels to avoid putting extra pressure on your legs.

Herbal remedies for varicose veins abound. Witch hazel applied directly to the skin at the site of the varicose vein can provide some temporary relief. Ginkgo biloba extract helps improve blood circulation and sometimes helps varicose veins. A traditional herbal remedy that is popular in Europe is made from horse chestnuts (also known as Ohio buckeye). Although horse chestnut extracts and tinctures are approved for use in Europe, they are not available in the United States. Another popular and moderately effective European herb for varicose veins is butcher's broom. Capsules containing butcher's broom are available in the U.S.; the usual dose is 325 milligrams twice daily. A number of other herbs, including vervain, hawthorn berry, white oak bark, and calendula are sometimes suggested by herbalists. None of these, however, is likely to affect your varicose veins.

Venous telangiectasia, spidery webs of blood vessels that appear on your thighs, are more of a cosmetic problem than a medical one. Elevating your legs can help.

❖ Yeast Infections

Once you've had one, there's no mistaking the symptoms of vaginal yeast infection: moderate to intense itching, an odorless white discharge that resembles cottage cheese, redness and swelling in the vaginal area, vaginal soreness, and a burning sensation, especially during intercourse. Almost every woman gets a yeast infection at some time in her life.

Yeast infections are usually caused by a fungus called *Candida albicans*. This organism is found normally in the vagina, but under certain conditions it can start to grow rapidly, resulting in a yeast infection. Some causes include normal hormonal changes, antibiotics, douching, pregnancy, diabetes, some kinds of birth control pills and spermicides, and being sweaty for long periods. Some unfortunate women seem to get yeast infections for no particular reason at all.

If you've never had a yeast infection before, see your doctor for a firm diagnosis. Yeast infections usually respond well to treatment with nonprescription antifungal medicines containing either clotrimazole or miconazole nitrate.

Diluted tea tree oil applied to the area can help relieve the itchiness of yeast infections. Calendula oil is a traditional herbal remedy that seems to help some women.

If you get frequent yeast infections, there are some practical steps you can take to avoid recurrences. Wear all-cotton underpants during the day, and skip underpants altogether at night. Avoid wearing tight trousers, panty hose, leggings, bathing suits, leotards, biking shorts, and other tightly fitting apparel for long periods. Whenever possible, wear loose clothing made from natural fabrics. Also avoid feminine hygiene products such as deodorants or douches, after-bath powders containing talc or cornstarch, bubble baths, colored toilet paper, and scented tampons. If you suspect that your birth control method is causing the problem, discuss alternatives with your doctor.

A preventive measure that seems to work for many women is eating a cup of plain, live-culture yogurt every day. Most supermarket yogurt does not contain live acidophilus bacteria. Try your health food store instead. If you don't like yogurt, try taking lactobacillus tablets. Do not put yogurt in your vagina.

See also Vaginitis.

❖
Healing
Herbs
❖

❖ Agrimony

Agrimonia spp.

Valued since the fifteenth century for its astringent properties, agrimony is traditionally recommended for external use to treat skin inflammations, pimples, cuts, and scrapes. It is also said to help stem bleeding from cuts, relieve itchy insect bites, and soothe athlete's foot. Gargling with a mild infusion of agrimony can ease a sore throat. Agrimony's high silica content may account for its tissue-healing abilities. People with very sensitive skin should apply agrimony with caution, as it has been known to cause allergic reactions.

Herbalists sometimes suggest using an agrimony eyewash to treat conjunctivitis. However, this is not a good idea. Never use herbal products in your eyes.

❖ Alfalfa

Medicago sativa

Alfalfa, a member of the legume (bean) family, is low in calories and fat and high in the B vitamins, vitamin C, vitamin K, carotene, chlorophyll, and eight essential enzymes.

A good source of biotin, calcium, iron, and protein, alfalfa also contains natural fluoride, which helps prevent tooth decay. For years, the only place to find alfalfa sprouts was in health food stores, but now they're available in the produce section of most supermarkets. You can even buy alfalfa seeds and sprout them yourself. Juicing the sprouts is a tasty way to get a good portion of your daily vitamins and minerals.

Although alfalfa is a great health food for most people, avoid it if you have the autoimmune disorder lupus. The amino acid L-canavanine found in alfalfa can make lupus symptoms worse.

❖ Aloe

Aloe vera

Aloe, a fleshy, perennial plant, was known to the ancient Greeks for its healing qualities. Today, this easily grown houseplant is still valued as a veritable first aid kit. To relieve the pain of a minor burn or cut, break off a piece from one of the plant's thick leaves and rub the plant's gel on the affected area. Aloe gel is also an effective treatment for minor sunburns and dry skin.

Stabilized aloe gel, which is said to have the same healing properties as the fresh gel, is listed as an ingredient in many commercial creams, ointments, and other products. Not all of these products are what they claim, however. Some actually contain aloe that is made from aloe extract or reconstituted aloe. Others contain so little aloe that they are very unlikely to be effective. For best results, keep an aloe vera plant on the kitchen windowsill.

Aloe juice, not gel, is used by some people as a purgative to treat constipation. Aloe juice or powdered aloe is prepared from aloe leaves, but not from the gel secreted by the inner cells of the plants. Aloe juice comes from special cells found just below the outer rind of the leaves. Taken as a tincture or in capsules, aloe juice is a powerful purgative. Since there are far gentler and safer ways to relieve constipation, aloe juice should not be used.

❖ Angelica

Angelica spp.

According to Christian folklore, during a plague in the Middle Ages, the Archangel Michael taught a monk how to use the curative powers of this plant. From that day forward, the plant always bloomed on May 8, the Feast of St. Michael, and so was named in his honor.

In Western herbal lore, *Angelica archangelica* is the variety most commonly used. Native to northern regions, the plant grows to be 5 to 8 feet tall. It prefers a shady environment with moist, rich soil. With wide, hollow stems and a leafy top, angelica looks a bit like a giant celery. All parts of the angelica plant contain a highly aromatic oil that has an aniselike aroma. An important ingredient in the secret formulas used to make the liqueurs Benedictine and Chartreuse, it's also used in baking, potpourris, and even some perfumes. The stems are sometimes candied and eaten as a confection.

Angelica tea is traditionally recommended as a treatment for coughing from colds or bronchitis. Although there is no scientific proof that angelica relieves cough symptoms, some patients claim it is very effective.

Because angelica is reputed to regulate the menstrual flow and induce uterine contractions during labor (little medical evidence supports this), it was sometimes taken in large amounts in an attempt to induce abortion. Not only does this not work, it is potentially very dangerous. Angelica should be avoided by pregnant women.

Angelica contains a number of chemical compounds called psoralens, which can increase the sensitivity of your skin to light. For this reason, many doctors advise against eating angelica candy, since it can cause a type of dermatitis that can lead to skin cancer. Psoralens are sometimes effective for treating psoriasis and some other skin conditions. However, do not attempt to treat psoriasis yourself with any form of angelica.

One final word of warning: Angelica strongly resembles water hemlock, a very poisonous plant. Don't collect angelica yourself—buy it only from a reputable source.

See also Dong Quai.

❖ Anise

Pimpinella anisum

Whether prescribed by Hippocrates as a cough medicine, traded as currency, used as an aphrodisiac, or put under your pillow to ward off bad dreams, anise has always been a valued herb. A member of the same family as celery and carrots, anise prefers a hot, dry, sunny environment. The licoricelike flavor of anise is commercially used to flavor everything from liqueurs to toothpaste. Although the leaves contain some flavor, the seeds contain the most aromatic oils. Ground anise is an often-used flavoring in baking and in Chinese cooking (it's one of the essential ingredients in five-spice powder). The Romans used to bake a special anise cake that was served at the end of a feast. Aside from tasting delicious, they believed the anise aided digestion.

In herbal lore, anise is still recommended as a digestive aid. Taken before meals, aniseed tea is considered to be a mild appetite stimulant. The tea is also said to help relieve gas, bloating, nausea, and indigestion. A few drops in a baby's bottle are said to help relieve gas and colic. Aniseed tea is also traditionally recommended to nursing mothers to help promote milk production, although it is probably the additional liquid, not the anise, that helps. For a natural breath freshener, try chewing a few aniseeds.

❖ Apple

Malus spp.

The original health food, apples are low in calories, fat, and sodium, high in fiber, and have only about 80 calories apiece. An excellent source of the trace mineral boron, which is needed for healthy bones, one medium-sized apple provides about a third of your daily requirement. More than 80 percent of the fiber in an apple is water-soluble pectin, the type of fiber credited with helping to lower blood cholesterol levels. Pectin can also help prevent constipation and relieve diarrhea symptoms. In fact, many doctors suggest eating applesauce or grated apples to help ease a bout of intestinal flu. Apple juice, on the other hand, has even higher levels of pectin, which can give some people, especially children, mild diarrhea.

❖ Arnica

Arnica spp.

An herb in the aster family, arnica has an orange, daisylike flower. As Europeans and Native Americans discovered independently of each other centuries ago, arnica flowers, made into a tincture or ointment, can relieve the discomfort of bruises, sprains, and muscular aches and pains when rubbed into the skin at the affected area. Today, a wide range of arnica creams, ointments, tinctures, and other preparations are available. Of these, tinctures are the most effective, though perhaps the least convenient.

Arnica should be used externally only, and then only on unbroken skin. Arnica tablets are sometimes recommended by herbalists and homeopathic practitioners, but these can cause dangerous increases in blood pressure and other symptoms of poisoning. Arnica should not be used internally.

❖ Astragalus

Astragalus membranaceus
In traditional Chinese medicine, astragalus (also called huang qi or huang chi) is recommended for persistent or frequent colds, fatigue, and infections. It is said to improve immune system function and increase your production of white blood cells. It has a mild diuretic effect and is also said to protect the liver and relieve depression. The root is generally used in a decoction or tincture; sometimes the root is powdered and taken in capsules.

❖ Balm

Melissa officinalis
A fragrant woodland herb, balm (also sometimes called lemon balm or melissa) is purported to renew youth and to stave off senility and impotency—practically an elixir of life. Needless to say, these claims are more than a little ex-

aggerated. Balm does have a pleasant, lemon-mint scent and makes an enjoyable herbal tea, which is often recommended for its calming effect. It's also said to aid digestion.

Balm shows significant promise as a treatment for cold sores caused by the herpes virus. In Europe, an ointment containing concentrated lemon balm extract is prescribed for herpes simplex infections, including cold sores and genital herpes. Applying the ointment regularly seems to help the sores heal faster and cut back on recurrences. Although balm ointment is not available in the United States, herpes sufferers could try making a strong infusion of the herb by steeping 1 tablespoon of finely chopped leaves in 1/2 cup of boiling water for ten minutes. Soak some cotton balls in the cooled solution and hold them against the sores for a few minutes; repeat several times a day.

❖ Banana

Musa sapientum

Technically speaking a banana is an herb because it is part of the flower made by the female banana plant. To confuse matters even more, botanically speaking, the banana is a berry—a fleshy fruit that develops from a single plant ovary and has few seeds. Be that as it may, most people think of a banana as a delicious fruit that comes in its own convenient wrapping.

Many doctors suggest eating bananas if you have diarrhea. They're easy to digest, nutritious, and won't further irritate your bowels. The pectin in the bananas helps relieve diarrhea symptoms, and it may also help protect you against colon cancer. Eating bananas often relieves the symptoms of nauseous indigestion and may also help heal gastric ulcers. Because bananas are fairly bland and easy to mash, they go down easily if you have a sore throat and trouble swallowing.

❖ Barberry

Mahonia spp.; formerly known as *Berberis vulgaris*

Also known as Oregon grape, barberry was used by the Native Americans as an appetite stimulant and general tonic. Herbalists recommend it as an astringent tea to relieve diarrhea symptoms; gargling with barberry tea can relieve the discomfort of a sore throat. Barberry contains a number of medicinally active alkaloid compounds. One compound, berberine, was once prescribed by physicians as a heart tonic and as a treatment for bronchial spasms, but for decades far more effective and safer drugs have been available. Another compound in barberry, berbamine, can lower blood pressure. If you have high blood pressure, however, do not attempt to treat it yourself with barberry—see your doctor.

❖ Basil

Ocimum spp.

Basil has been used as a medicinal and aromatic herb for thousands of years. In its native India, basil is considered a sacred herb; an infusion of basil is used in burial rites. In Ayurvedic medicine, basil juice is used as a treatment for coughs, skin problems, and as a general tonic. Basil was also recommended by the ancient Greek physicians as a treatment for stomach upsets, coughs, and nervous conditions. A snuff made from basil was used as a headache remedy in colonial America. In Asia, basil has been used as a cough medicine. Modern aromatherapy uses basil oil to ease depression, nervousness, and emotional fatigue. Because basil is related to mint, some herbalists suggest basil tea for easing heartburn and indigestion.

Today, basil has no real medicinal use, but it is increasingly popular in the kitchen. Sweet basil *(Ocimum basilicum)*, the most common form of basil, is widely used as an aromatic cooking herb, especially in tomato sauces. It's also the prime ingredient in pesto. As basil has gotten more popular, some exotic varieties have become available. Look for lettuce-leaf basil, Greek basil, lemon basil, and purple basil alongside sweet basil in the produce section.

Dried basil just doesn't have the same flavor as fresh leaves. Fortunately, a potted basil plant is very easy to grow indoors on a windowsill. It prefers a warm, sunny spot and rich, moist soil. To keep the plant blooming and bushy, wait until it has four to six sets of leaves, then pinch back the plant. For each set of leaves you pluck off, two stems will develop. Pinch off any flower heads that form.

❖ Bay Leaf (Laurel)

Laurus nobilis
Bay leaves, also called laurel, have a rich history. In Greek mythology, laurel leaves signified victory and merit—a symbolism we continue today in the terms *crown of laurels, poet laureate,* and *baccalaureate.* During the Middle Ages, people believed that bay leaves would protect them from witches and evil spirits and would ward off the plague. Modern herbalists sometimes suggest a tea made from bay leaves to relieve indigestion and gas. Bay leaf oil, available at health food stores, is sometimes suggested as a treatment for aching, arthritic joints. Rub the oil into the skin above the affected area. To soothe aching muscles, try soaking in a warm bath that contains a strong bay infusion.

Today, bay leaves are more likely to be found in the kitchen than in the medicine chest. Look for bay leaves with slightly wavy edges; these come from Mediterranean laurel trees. Smooth-edged leaves are probably from the California laurel and will be less flavorful. One of three ingredients of the classic French bouquet garni, bay is a wonderful flavoring for hearty soups, stews, and sauces. It takes some time for bay to release its flavor, so add it at the beginning of a recipe. Bay leaves remain tough even after cooking and must be removed from the dish before serving. Here's a useful pantry tip: A bay leaf in the flour canister helps ward off bugs.

Be very careful when picking laurel in the wild. Some plants with laurel in their name, such as mountain laurel, are poisonous. Only *Laurus nobilis* is edible.

❖ Bayberry

Myrica pensylvanica

A low, shrubby plant that thrives in poor, sandy soil, bayberry has small, blue white berries. The berries contain a fragrant, waxy substance that today is often used to scent candles, bath oils, and soap. In earlier times, bayberry bark was used as a treatment for diarrhea; it was thought to be effective because of the bark's high tannin content. That same high tannin level, however, makes bayberry potentially carcinogenic. Enjoy bayberry's aroma, but don't take it internally.

❖ Bee Balm

Monarda didyma

An American native, bee balm was used by Indians as a medicinal tea. Colonial settlers also drank it, sometimes calling it Oswego tea after the tribe that introduced it to them. Bee balm was said to help the digestion and relieve gas as well as menstrual discomfort, but its chief virtue seems to have been its mild, lemony flavor. Enjoy bee balm as a refreshing herbal tea, but don't expect any medicinal value from it. Today, bee balm is grown primarily as an ornamental plant in the garden. The tubular shape of its brilliant scarlet flowers makes it irresistible to hummingbirds.

❖ Bee Pollen

The golden dust gathered from the stamen of flowers by bees, bee pollen has enjoyed some sensational press, especially once it became known that members of Great Britain's royal family were using it. Some natural medicine practitioners and nutritionists claim that bee pollen can enhance your vitality and improve your immune system function. Bee pollen contains 185 nutrients (including twenty-two amino acids), a full array of vitamins (including a good amount of vitamin B_{12}), and many minerals such as calcium, iron, and potassium. It's possible that a daily spoonful or two could give you the vitamins and minerals you need just as well as a multivitamin tablet. Proponents of bee pollen claim that it fights fatigue, depression, and has an antimicrobial effect, although there isn't a lot of medical evidence to support this. Some people who are allergic to pollen may be allergic to bee pollen. Stop taking it if you develop a rash, wheeze, get hives, or have any other related symptoms.

❖ Betony

Stachys officinalis

In the centuries it has been used as a medicinal herb, betony (also called wood betony) has been recommended for just

about every ailment there is, not to mention its supposed value
for warding off evil spirits. Today, betony's medicinal uses are
confined to treating diarrhea and minor throat and mouth irritation. The high tannin content of this herb helps relieve diarrhea symptoms when it is taken as a tea. The astringent effect
of the tannin soothes sore throats and mouth irritation; use it as
a gargle or rinse. Betony also contains glycosides, which can
lower your blood pressure, but this is not an effective treatment. If you have high blood pressure, see your doctor.

Betony makes an attractive garden plant because of its
showy flower spikes. Use the leaves and stems to make tea.

❖ Bilberry
See Blueberry.

❖ Birch

Betula spp.
The bark and leaves of both the silver and the white birch
are important in Native American herbal lore. The bark was
made into a tea said to relieve headaches, fever, and muscle
cramps. Tea made from the leaves was said to have a diuretic effect. As is often the case, traditional wisdom is well-
founded. Because birch contains methyl salicylate, a
substance similar to aspirin, there may be some validity to
its use for pain and fever. Birch leaves have been approved
in Germany for use as a diuretic. However, discuss using
birch leaves as a diuretic with your doctor before trying
them.

❖ Black Cohosh

Cimicifuga racemosa

Long valued by Native Americans as a remedy for many ailments, particularly those related to menstruation, black cohosh is also sometimes called black snakeroot. Later, black cohosh was an important ingredient in patent medicines recommended for "women's troubles." Recent research has revealed the scientific basis for the folkloric wisdom—extracts made from the dried root and rhizomes contain substances that do help relieve premenstrual stress (PMS), painful menstruation, and some menopause symptoms. In particular, black cohosh can reduce the number and duration of hot flashes by reducing the amount of luteinizing hormone produced by a menopausal woman. Do not use black cohosh if you are pregnant or think you might be.

In Germany, an alcoholic extract of black cohosh is approved for use as a treatment for PMS, dysmenorrhea, and some menopause symptoms. The usual dose is several teaspoons a day. In tea form, an equivalent dose could be made by steeping 3 teaspoons of powdered root in 1/2 cup of boiling water for ten minutes. Strain before drinking. Not much is known about the long-term effects of using black cohosh, however, so discuss this herb with your doctor before trying it.

❖ Black Currant

Ribes nigrum

Both the leaves and the fruit of the European black currant bush are used in traditional herbal medicine. Black currant fruit was said to be a good remedy for kidney ailments, and a tea made of the leaves or the juice from the berries was said to stimulate the kidneys and increase urine flow. Today, black currant oil is of great interest to researchers because it is very high in gamma-linolenic acid (GLA), the same substance found in evening primrose oil. Since many herbalists and natural medicine practitioners claim that GLA can affect myriad health problems, ranging from weight loss to multiple sclerosis, black currant oil capsules are now sold in health food stores. However, little evidence supports the claims that GLA has any medicinal value.

See also Evening Primrose Oil.

❖ Black Hellebore

Helliborus niger

This winter-blooming perennial is sometimes grown as an ornamental. Although black hellebore is sometimes used in homeopathic medicine in very small doses, it is highly poisonous and should never be ingested. Even touching the leaves can cause contact dermatitis for some people. If you have small children and this plant grows in your garden, consider removing it to avoid accidents.

❖ Black Pepper

Piper nigrum

The pepper plant, native to India, produces a small, berry-like fruit—the peppercorn. Today, pepper is inexpensive and everywhere, but centuries ago it was a rare and exotic Eastern spice imported to Europe at great cost. Not surprisingly, in those days pepper was often used as a medicine for a variety of ailments. Today, it has no medicinal uses at all.

❖ Blackberry

See Raspberry Leaves.

❖ Blessed Thistle

Cnicus benedictus

The leaves and stems of blessed thistle, a member of the aster family, are sometimes made into a tea and used as an appetite stimulant. The slightly bitter, astringent taste increases the flow of saliva and gastric juices, which makes you feel hungry.

❖ Bloodroot

Sanguinaria canadensis

Bloodroot, also called sanguinaria, gets its very apt name from its red-orange sap. A plant native to North America, bloodroot was used by Native Americans as a dye and as a medicine. In particular, bloodroot was noted as an expectorant that was particularly helpful for relieving lung congestion from bronchitis and flu. Native Americans also supposedly used bloodroot successfully to treat cancer, but there is little evidence that this is truly effective. The alkaloids found in bloodroot are quite potent, however, and bloodroot should not be used for self-treating any ailment.

Today, the only medically valid use for bloodroot is as an ingredient in commercially prepared natural toothpastes and mouthwashes. It has been shown to be safe and effective for helping to prevent plaque and gum disease. Because bloodroot can be toxic, do not attempt to prepare your own homemade dental products with it.

Blue Cohosh

Caulophyllum thalictroides

Although herbalists often recommend blue cohosh for many of the same ailments as black cohosh, these two plants are completely different and should not be confused. Today, it is usually suggested as a treatment for menstrual difficulties. However, blue cohosh contains caulosaponin, a powerful glycoside that can raise blood pressure, cause intestinal spasms, and constrict the blood vessels leading to the heart. This herb is potentially dangerous and should not be used for any purpose.

❖ Blueberry

Vaccinium corymbosum (American) or *Vaccinium myrtillus* (European)

Both the leaves and the fruit of the blueberry plant have useful medicinal value. One of the few foods that are naturally blue in color, the blueberry and its close European cousin, the bilberry, contain large amounts of a complex organic compound called anthocyanoside. In concentrated form, this compound has been shown to help slow vision loss due to macular degeneration.

Botanically speaking, blueberries and cranberries are closely related. Cranberry juice has been shown to help prevent bladder infections in women, and blueberries can have the same effect. The reason is that both berries contain a substance that blocks infection-causing bacteria from adhering to the bladder. Blueberries are also a good source of dietary fiber, largely in the form of pectin. This soluble fiber may help protect you against colon cancer and can help lower your blood cholesterol levels.

Dried blueberry leaves are high in tannin, and tea made from the leaves can help relieve diarrhea. Dried (not fresh) blueberries are a traditional European remedy for diarrhea. Soak a teaspoonful or so of the berries in 1 cup boiling water until the berries are softened, about five minutes. Drink the liquid and then eat the berries. Repeat three to seven times daily. The tannins and pectin in the blueberries make this remedy effective. Tea made from dried blueberry leaves can also be effective for diarrhea because of the high tannin content. Use 1 or 2 teaspoons of leaves to 1 cup boiling water. Let steep for ten to fifteen minutes before drinking.

❖ Boneset

Eupatorium perfoliatum
Boneset, a member of the daisy family, was brewed into a tea by Native Americans and early colonists and used as a treatment for colds and flu. Although some modern-day herbalists still recommend boneset, no evidence has shown that it has any beneficial effect whatsoever. In fact, the tea

has an extremely bitter and unpleasant taste that often nauseates patients and leads to vomiting.

❖ Borage

Borago officinalis

From the first century onward, borage has been recommended for inducing courage, lifting depression, increasing urination, and relieving sore throats—presumably not simultaneously. Despite its long history of use, borage hasn't been proven to do any of those things. The seeds of this hairy perennial plant, however, are a good source of gamma linolenic acid (GLA), the same substance found in evening primrose oil. Since many herbalists and natural medicine practitioners claim that GLA can help health problems such as psoriasis and multiple sclerosis, capsules containing borage seed oil are now sold in health food stores. There is little evidence, however, that GLA has any medicinal value.

Borage leaves, stems, and flowers have a taste that is slightly like cucumber. Sprigs of borage are sometimes added to flavor vinegar for salad dressings. Borage also flavors the mixed drink known as Pimm's Cup.

❖ Brewer's Yeast

Also sometimes called nutritional yeast, brewer's yeast is a brown powder made from the same one-celled organisms that are used to ferment beer. Because it is very high in protein and contains many vitamins (including most of the B vitamins), minerals, and amino acids, brewer's yeast is sometimes used as a food supplement, particularly by athletes. Herbalists and natural medicine practitioners often recommend it as an energy booster. The powder is usually taken in capsules or mixed with juice or water. Despite claims, there is little or no evidence that brewer's yeast can be effective for treating heart problems, diabetes, eczema, psoriasis, or gout. Neither will it keep fleas or mosquitoes away.

❖ Broom

Cytisus spp.
Once widely used in herbal medicine, broom is a dangerous herb that can cause fatal poisoning. Do not use it for any medicinal purpose. Do not confuse this herb with butcher's broom (see page 209).

❖ Buchu

Barosma spp.
Buchu leaves come from a small, South African shrub. The leaves contain a volatile oil that has a mild diuretic effect. Buchu is rather uncommon in the United States, but it is widely used in Europe in commercial herbal tea blends meant to treat bladder conditions.

❖ Buckthorn

Rhamnus spp.
Alder buckthorn, common buckthorn, and cascara sagrada (California buckthorn) are all used primarily for their laxa-

tive and diuretic effects. Buckthorn relieves constipation without irritating the system. It has strong purgative results, however, and should be used in small doses. A tonic made from the bark is used as a digestive aid. Buckthorn compresses are used to relieve minor skin irritations.

Pregnant women should avoid all forms of buckthorn. Bark must be aged for at least a year and berries should not be eaten in large quantities to avoid toxic effects.

See also Cascara Sagrada.

❖ Burdock

Arctium lappa

Burdock has long been a valued plant in herbal medicine. All parts of the plant are said to be useful, although the root is considered most valuable. Traditionally, burdock has been recommended for skin diseases, blood disorders, kidney troubles, chronic infections, gout, rheumatism, sciatica, indigestion, and constipation. Since there is nothing in burdock that actually has any effect on any of these ailments, burdock's reputation is very puzzling.

Burdock root is a mainstay of macrobiotic diets. It is a fairly good dietary source of iron, copper, zinc, and manganese. Purchase your burdock from a reliable vendor. The root looks a lot like the root of the poisonous belladonna plant.

❖ Butcher's Broom

Ruscus aculeatus

Not to be confused with broom (see entry on page 207), butcher's broom is a shrubby plant native to the Mediterranean region. Butcher's broom contains compounds that have an anti-inflammatory and vasoconstricting effect. Because of this, butcher's broom is a popular European remedy for hemorrhoids and varicose veins. Capsules containing butcher's broom are available in the United States; the usual dose for varicose veins is 325 milligrams twice daily. For hemorrhoids, use butcher's broom in ointment or suppository form. In either case, discuss using this herb with your doctor before you try it.

❖ Calendula (Pot Marigold)

Calendula officinalis

Calendula is a small plant with golden flowers that many people grow in window boxes and in gardens for its beauty. Although calendula's petals and essential oil have a rich tradition as cures for a wide range of diseases, today calendula's use is limited to herbal remedies for minor skin problems.

Although there is no real scientific basis for its effectiveness, calendula ointment does seem to help soothe minor cuts, scrapes, and skin irritations when applied externally. Try adding calendula oil to your bathwater to soften and soothe dry or slightly sunburned skin.

❖ Canaigre

Rumex hymenosepalus

A plant native to the deserts of the American southwest, canaigre root is sometimes sold under the names red American ginseng or desert ginseng. Touted as having a wide range of beneficial effects similar or superior to those of ginseng, in fact canaigre has no relation to ginseng at all. In addition, its high tannin content makes it potentially carcinogenic. Do not use canaigre in any form, as an alternative to ginseng or for any other reason.

See also Ginseng.

❖ Caraway

Carum carvi

Caraway seeds may have been used as long ago as the Stone Age to add flavors to foods, and the seeds have been found in Egyptian tombs. The pungent flavor is still popular today, especially in seeded rye bread.

Caraway seeds can be chewed to freshen your breath. In traditional herbal medicine, an infusion of caraway seeds is recommended as an aid to digestion. The seeds seem to have antispasmodic properties that calm the digestive tract. They also help relieve intestinal gas. An old—and often effective—folk remedy for gas and colic in babies is to put a few drops of caraway infusion into their bottle. Caraway may also help relax the uterine muscles—some women swear by its powers to relieve menstrual cramps. Although it is sometimes recommended to promote milk production in nursing mothers, pregnant women should avoid caraway.

❖ Cardamom

Elettaria cardamomum

Cardamom seeds, an aromatic spice used widely in Indian cooking as an ingredient in curry powder, also has some traditional medicinal uses. In India and China, cardamom seeds are chewed as an aid to digestion and for relieving nausea and flatulence. Chewing the seeds also freshens your breath naturally.

❖ Carrot

Daucus carota

Beta-carotene and fiber are found in abundance in carrots. Beta-carotene, the precursor to vitamin A, is one of the most effective antioxidants. Aside from its protective powers against cancer and heart disease, beta-carotene promotes healthy eyes and good night vision, and protects you against cataracts and macular degeneration. Beta-carotene can also give your immune system a boost, helping you to fend off infections. A single raw carrot gives you some 11,000 IU of vitamin A (which includes beta-carotene), or more than 250 percent of the recommended dietary allowance. And carrots also contain water-soluble fiber, which has been shown to help reduce blood cholesterol levels. One raw carrot has about 1 gram of fiber and only about 40 calories. Many people claim that carrot juice helps their digestion, relieving the discomfort of heartburn and gas.

Wild carrots must be gathered with caution because there are poisonous plants that look just like the edible kinds. Vitamin A can be toxic when ingested in large quantities, so be careful not to overdo it.

❖ Cascara Sagrada

Rhamnus purshiana

The dried bark of a small tree found in the Pacific Northwest, cascara sagrada can be used as a mild laxative. Its beneficial effects come from the anthraquinones in the bark. To reduce the concentration of these powerful chemicals and prevent unpleasant side effects, cascara sagrada bark should be aged for at least a year before it is used. Over-the-counter preparations of the bark are usually in the form of a liquid extract with some flavoring added to disguise the extremely bitter taste. The usual dosage is very small—just 1/2 teaspoon is effective. Capsules and pills containing the powdered bark are also available.

Another laxative herb, buckthorn, is botanically very similar to cascara sagrada but comes from a shrub found in Europe and eastern Asia. Its effects and use are virtually the same.

❖ Castor Bean

Ricinus communis

A popular ornamental plant, the castor bean is the source of castor oil, a mild but foul-tasting laxative. The seeds containing the oil also contain a dangerous chemical called ricin that can cause vomiting, diarrhea, and blurred vision. Small children can die from eating just a single seed. Use castor oil only on the advice of your doctor. For safety's sake, don't grow castor beans in a garden frequented by young children.

❖ Catnip

Nepeta cataria

Cat lovers the world over know the magical effect that cat-nip has on their furry friends, but many don't realize the plant's effects on humans. While catnip gets kitty all revved up, it has the opposite effect on people. Tea made from cat-nip leaves has a pleasant lemon-minty flavor. It acts as a very mild natural sedative that can soothe your nerves and help you fall asleep. Its relaxing properties may offer relief from headaches and menstrual cramps. Catnip, a member of the mint family, is a traditional herbal remedy for stomach upsets, colic, and intestinal gas. The leaf and flower contain some vitamin C, so its traditional use as a remedy for sore throats, fever, and the common cold may have some scien-tific basis.

❖ Cayenne Pepper (Chili Pepper, Hot Pepper)

Capsicum annuum

Technically speaking, cayenne (hot) peppers are berries, the fruit of shrubs in the *Capsicum* genus. A single hot pepper contains a full day's supply of beta-carotene and nearly twice the recommended dietary allowance for vitamin C. (Bell peppers and paprika, sweet members of the *Capsicum* genus, also have large amounts of these vitamins.)

Hot peppers get their bite from a compound called cap-saicin. When applied to the skin, capsaicin can block pain impulses. For this reason, ointments containing capsaicin are used to relieve the pain of shingles; they have also been used to some effect for treating psoriasis and arthritis. Capsaicin can help lower your LDL (bad) blood cholesterol and reduce your triglyceride levels and may also keep your blood from forming the dangerous clots that could lead to a heart attack or stroke. The capsaicin in hot peppers can also help clear up stuffy noses and congested bronchial tubes. Hot peppers help stimulate gastric juices, so they act as an effective appetite stimulant as well as add flavorful spiciness to food. Despite popular misconceptions, hot peppers do not cause ulcers or gallbladder problems.

❖ Celery

Apium graveolens

In many cultures, celery is used as a traditional remedy for high blood pressure. Until recently, modern doctors had recommended against using it this way, citing the high sodium level. Studies show, however, that celery, despite its sodium content, contains a chemical that reduces the blood pressure in laboratory animals. (It also lowered the animals' cholesterol levels.) Two to four ribs of celery a day would be the human equivalent to the dosage the laboratory animals received. Celery has a lot of sodium for a vegetable, but the amount it contains is still quite low—only about 35 milligrams a stalk—as compared with other foods. Celery is also a good source of fiber, vitamin A, and potassium. A single stalk has only about 20 calories.

Celery is a mild diuretic that can be helpful for relieving mild water retention and breast tenderness from premenstrual stress (PMS) symptoms. Celery also contains psoralens, compounds that may help relieve psoriasis symptoms.

❖ Chamomile

***Matricaria recutita* (German or Hungarian) or *Chamaemelum nobile,* formerly *Anthemis nobilis* (Roman or English)**

Two different but closely related herbs are called chamomile. Of the two, *Matricaria recutita,* better known as German or Hungarian chamomile, is the variety most commonly grown and used, especially in North America. Chamomile is an annual plant with small, daisylike flowers that have a faint scent of apple. Chamomile flowers have been used as a popular folk remedy for centuries.

When taken as a strong tea, chamomile can soothe upset stomachs, nausea, and heartburn. Many women claim it relieves menstrual cramps; it is also said to be good for relieving headaches. Chamomile tea is also effective for relieving minor mouth and gum irritation; use it as a mouthwash. (Steer clear of chamomile if you are allergic to ragweed, since you may be allergic to chamomile as well.) When applied externally as an extract or compress, chamomile helps alleviate swelling, inflammation, and minor skin irritations. A handful of chamomile flowers added to your bathwater softens and refreshes dry skin, provides soothing relief from sunburn, or creates a calming time-out after a stress-filled day. Cold chamomile tea is a wonderful hair rinse for blonds and redheads, enhancing highlights and conditioning hair at the same time, and it is used in many commercial shampoos and conditioners. Chamomile oil, which has a lovely blue color, is sometimes used as a massage oil. Some people find that rubbing chamomile oil into the skin at the site of an arthritic joint helps relieve pain. Some words of warning: Chamomile oil is a uterine stimulant and should be avoided during pregnancy. Most chamomile oil is imported from Europe. Since it is easy to adulterate this expensive oil, purchase only brands made by reputable companies.

Prepackaged chamomile tea bags are readily available at supermarkets everywhere. However, chamomile is often combined with other herbs, so check the listed ingredients. You can usually buy loose chamomile flowers (avoid powdered or crushed chamomile or flowers that have a lot of stems) at health food stores.

See also Yarrow.

❖ Chapparal

Larrea tridentata
Also called greasewood and creosote bush, chapparal is a scrubby shrub with a strong aroma. It is found widely throughout the desert regions of the Southwest. The Native Americans of the region used chapparal as a remedy for a wide variety of ailments, ranging from dandruff to snakebite. Similarly, modern-day herbalists recommend chapparal for a range of illnesses, claiming that the nordihydroguaiaretic acid (NDGA) it contains acts as an antibiotic and antioxidant. However, large doses of NDGA have been shown to be toxic and carcinogenic. The Food and Drug Administration removed chapparal from its list of herbs generally recognized as safe in 1968. Do not use chapparal for any medicinal or other purpose.

❖ Cherry

Prunus spp.
There are two types of cherries: sweet (popular varieties include bing, black, Windsor, and Napoleon, to name a few), and sour (known as tart, pie, or red cherries). These stone

fruits reach their peak availability between May and August, although chewy dried cherries are available year round. Fresh sweet cherries weigh in at only five calories each (or about 140 calories a cup). Furthermore, recent research shows that cherries contain a substance known as ellagic acid, an antioxidant compound that helps keep your cells from becoming cancerous. Cherries also have been linked to lower uric acid levels (useful if you have gout), and may be effective in their ability to help prevent collagen destruction. On average, water-soluble dietary fiber contributes 2.29 percent of the total weight of cherries. They're also a good source of vitamin A and potassium.

❖ Chickweed

Stellaria media
One of the most common and troublesome weeds to gardeners all over the world, chickweed is nonetheless widely recommended as an herbal remedy for just about anything. In particular, poultices made from chickweed are said to help heal skin irritations, cuts, scrapes, insect bites, boils, and so on. Despite its reputation, chickweed has no medicinal value whatsoever.

❖ Chives

Allium schoenoprasum
Bits of the thin, wispy leaf of the chive plant are often found sprinkled atop a sour cream–laden baked potato or mixed

with cream cheese for a tangy spread. But this cousin to onions and garlic has been a popular folk remedy for centuries. In fact, early Europeans believed it would chase away evil spirits and disease. As a member of the *Allium* genus, chives offer most of the health benefits of onions and garlic, but with a milder flavor.

See also Garlic; Onions.

❖ Cilantro
See Coriander.

❖ Cinnamon

Cinnamomum spp.
The aromatic, reddish brown spice sold in the United States as cinnamon might actually be from another, closely related plant called cassia. Both spices come from trees in the laurel family. The spice made from the dried bark of cassia is somewhat less expensive than genuine cinnamon, and both varieties are sold in various forms: as bark, ground powder, essential oil, or, in the case of cassia, dried buds.

In traditional Chinese medicine, cinnamon is said to have warming properties that are valuable for treating "cold" conditions such as kidney ailments. In Western herbal medicine, cinnamon is used for relieving the symptoms of a variety of minor illnesses. Tea made from cinnamon bark is sometimes helpful for relieving nausea, heartburn, and indigestion; it's also good for cold symptoms. If you have a cough and stuffy nose, try adding a few drops of cinnamon oil to boiling water and inhale the steam. Cinnamon oil also makes a warming and aromatic addition to massage oil. A few drops are all you need. Some people claim that cinnamon oil is effective as an antiseptic for minor cuts and skin irritations; others say it works well as an antifungal for athlete's foot. Use cinnamon oil cautiously, however. It may cause redness and burning if applied directly to the skin, and can cause nausea, vomiting, and possible kidney damage if ingested. Cinnamon in general is a uterine stimulant, so avoid medicinal amounts during pregnancy.

❖ Cloves

Syzygium aromaticum

Cloves are the dried flower buds of an evergreen tree found originally in the tropical regions of the Indian Ocean. The sharp fragrance of cloves makes them a good natural breath freshener; try sticking a handful of buds directly into an orange for a natural, air-freshening pomander. The familiar smell of cloves is found in many commercial shampoos, soaps, and perfumes. As a cooking spice, cloves are widely used to flavor baked goods, stews, soups, pickles, marinades, and mulled drinks, among many other foods.

Medicinally, the most familiar and widespread use of cloves is as a temporary remedy for toothache. In an emergency, you can temporarily relieve the discomfort of a toothache with clove oil. Soak a cotton ball in the oil and rub it directly against the aching tooth and gums. Clove oil is also used to flavor many toothpastes and mouthwashes. Clove tea is an old folk remedy for indigestion and nausea. In traditional Chinese herbal medicine, cloves are used to treat indigestion, diarrhea, ringworm, athlete's foot, and fungal infections.

Although cloves contain antioxidants, which help prevent cell damage that can lead to cancer, they also contain eugenol, a chemical that is a weak tumor promoter. Cancer patients should probably avoid cloves. Note that clove cigarettes are not safer than tobacco cigarettes. Tobacco comprises at least half of the ingredients in a clove cigarette, and cloves release many carcinogens when burned.

❖ Coffee

Coffea arabica

A passion for some people, an addiction for others, coffee has spawned quite a bit of controversy over the last few years. The controversy revolves around the caffeine found in coffee and its effect on the human body. At various times caffeine has been linked to heart disease, bladder cancer, breast cancer, birth defects, and other diseases. In fact, there is no evidence that drinking coffee causes heart disease, cancer, high blood pressure, osteoporosis, high cholesterol, or any other serious ailment.

Caffeine is part of a group of naturally occurring compounds called methylxanthines. They're found in coffee beans, cola nuts, tea leaves, cocoa beans, and maté, a South American herbal drink. Caffeine stimulates the central nervous system. In some people, even small amounts can cause insomnia. In large amounts, it can cause nervousness, headaches, anxiety, irritability, and a slight rise in blood pressure. Caffeine is absorbed into the bloodstream within a few minutes and excreted in the urine in about three hours. The effects, however, vary from individual to individual.

In general, coffee is a safe and effective mild stimulant. A cup or two makes most people feel more alert and awake; a quiet cup of coffee often helps relieve mild headaches. If caffeine keeps you from sleeping, avoid it for at least three hours before bedtime. If you have high blood pressure or heart disease (particularly any problems with irregular heartbeats), discuss drinking coffee with your doctor. It is probably safe for you to have it in moderation (2 cups a day). Pregnant women are usually advised to avoid caffeine altogether, but recent studies suggest that a daily cup or two of coffee is not a problem. If you have gallstones or ulcers, it might be wise to avoid coffee—it could bring on an attack.

A 5-ounce brewed cup of coffee has about 115 milligrams of caffeine; a 5-ounce percolated cup has about 80 milligrams. (By comparison, a 5-ounce cup of brewed tea has 40 to 60 milligrams of caffeine.) Decaffeinated coffee is specially processed to remove about 97 percent of the caffeine. Caffeine may be extracted by minimal amounts of methylene chloride (a controversial substance which has been found to cause cancer when inhaled in large amounts by lab animals) or by ethyl acetate (a naturally occurring substance in fruits and vegetables.) Caffeine may also be removed by the Swiss water process. The coffee beans are steamed in water and the caffeine-containing outer layer is removed. Coffee flavor is determined by the type of bean used, the growing conditions (soil and climate), and how the bean was roasted. The darker the roast, the stronger the flavor.

❖ Coltsfoot

Tussilago farfara

Over the centuries, coltsfoot was often used as a treatment for coughs. One treatment had patients *smoking* the hoof-shaped green leaves for relief from asthma and coughing—an illogical practice that is certainly not recommended now. Today, herbalists still recommend coltsfoot tea for coughs and wheezing. The mucilage in the leaves may have a mildly soothing effect, but coltsfoot also contains an alkaloid substance that is a known liver carcinogen. Internal use of coltsfoot is not recommended.

However, applied as a poultice to minor scrapes, insect bites, burns, and skin irritations, coltsfoot leaves have a somewhat astringent and soothing effect.

❖ Comfrey

Symphytum officinale
Comfrey has been used as a healing herb at least since the days of ancient Greece. Simple casts to set broken bones were made on ancient battlefields by boiling comfrey and dipping cloth in the pasty residue. The cloth was then wrapped around the affected area; it dried to a plasterlike hardness.

Over the centuries, comfrey tea became a popular prescription for just about anything. It was used variously to treat diarrhea, colitis, dysentery, bronchitis, ulcers, and menstrual disorders. While some herbalists still endorse the internal use of comfrey, and many people use it as a gargle for throat inflammations, hoarseness, and bleeding gums, consumption of comfrey is definitely not recommended. Comfrey contains alkaloids that are known to cause liver disease and cancer and should never be taken internally.

However, comfrey does have some safe external uses. Because it contains allantoin, a substance that promotes the growth of new cells, comfrey poultices, creams, and ointments can help relieve inflammation and discomfort from minor skin irritations, bruising, and minor burns. (When applying comfrey leaves or root to any kind of wound, make sure that area and the herb have been thoroughly cleaned first.) A long soak in a comfrey bath is good for sore muscles and sunburned skin.

Some herbal reference books contain a recipe for a burn ointment made from comfrey, wheat germ oil, and honey. The mixture is smeared over the burn and left in place. It is said to feed the tissue, promote healing, and reduce scarring. In fact, this is a recipe for infection. If you have a burn severe enough to require treatment, see your doctor.

Comfrey root contains twice as much allantoin as the leaves. Unfortunately, the comfrey root strongly resembles the root of the poisonous water hemlock plant. Mix-ups have occurred. Purchase your comfrey only from a reliable source.

❖ Coriander (Cilantro)

Coriandrum sativum

The use of coriander has been mentioned in such diverse documents as ancient Sanskrit texts, *Tales of the Arabian Nights,* and the Bible (where manna was said to taste like coriander). Seeds have been found in Egyptian tombs, and it was used as a meat preservative in ancient Rome. In ancient China, India, and Europe in the Middle Ages it was thought to be an aphrodisiac. In Elizabethan times an aromatic coriander seed was used as the center of a hard candy, the precursor of our modern jawbreaker candies.

The pungent green leaves of coriander are also called cilantro or Chinese parsley; the dried ripe fruits are known as coriander seeds. Although their tastes are rather different, both the leaves and seeds are said to have similar healing effects. Chewing on coriander seeds or drinking a tea made from the leaves or seeds are traditional remedies for such digestive problems as gas, heartburn, diarrhea, and stomach pain. Because it is quite mild, a few drops of a weak infusion of the leaves or seeds can be given to babies for gas and colic.

❖ Corn Silk

Zea mays

Corn silk, the long, thin fibers found between the husk and the kernels on fresh ears of corn, is sometimes used as a mild diuretic. Herbalists often suggest corn silk tea to relieve painful urination from an enlarged prostrate. However, if you are experiencing painful urination for any reason, see your doctor.

❖ Couch Grass

Agropyrum repens

Couch grass (also sometimes called witch grass or quack grass) is a weedy perennial grass native to Europe and naturalized in many parts of the United States. Tea made from couch grass root is recommended by herbalists for kidney and bladder stones; drinking the tea is said to help patients pass stones. To make couch grass tea, use 1 teaspoon of root per cup of water; bring to a boil and let cool. Strain before drinking. The usual dose is 1 to 2 cups a day. If you have kidney or bladder stones or tend to get them, discuss using couch grass tea with your doctor before you try it.

❖ Cranberry

Vaccinium macrocarpon

Women who are prone to bladder infections have long known that cranberry juice helps relieve the symptoms, shortens the attack, and even prevents recurrences. Just why cranberry juice works was long a subject of debate. For years, doctors thought it was because the acidity of cranberry juice made the urine more acidic. Instead, recent studies show that cranberry juice inhibits the growth of harmful bacteria by keeping them from adhering to the lining of the bladder and urethra. If you think you have a urinary tract infection, see your doctor. Antibiotics will usually clear it up in just a day or so. If you get urinary tract infections often, having a daily glass of cranberry juice may reduce their frequency and severity. Fresh, unsweetened cranberry juice is the most effective and least caloric, but it is usually available only at health food stores. If the natural, unsweetened verion is too tart for you, mix it with apple, pear, or grape juices, or try capsules containing cranberry extract. The commercially prepared cranberry juice sold in supermarkets is often heavily sweetened with corn syrup and diluted somewhat with water, but it will still help urinary tract infections.

❖ Cucumber

Cucumis sativus

A vine vegetable that originated in India, cucumbers contain sterols, compounds that could help lower your blood cholesterol level. The occasional bitter taste of a cucumber is due to a compound known as cucurbitacin, which may have antitumor effects. In traditional Chinese herbal medicine, cucumber is prescribed to treat burns and laryngitis. The dark green skin contains most of the nutrients in a cucumber: traces of vitamins and minerals, along with silica, a mineral necessary for strong connective tissues. To reduce puffiness and revive tired eyes, try placing cool cucumber slices on your eyes.

❖ Damiana

Turnera diffusa, var. aphrodisiaca

The leaves of this Mexican shrub are said to be an aphrodisiac, although there is absolutely no scientific substantiation. Damiana supposedly stimulates the reproductive organs and promotes sexual drive, and is sometimes prescribed by herbalists for impotence, hormone imbalances, and menopausal problems. Mexican liqueurs containing tiny amounts of damiana are available: however, these do not contain enough of the herb to have any effect aside from flavoring. Despite what people say, drinking damiana tea or smoking dried damiana leaves won't have an aphrodisiac effect, either.

❖ Dandelion

Taraxacum officinale

Transported to the New World by European settlers, the leaves, stems, and roots of the ubiquitous dandelion have traditionally been considered a cure-all for a considerable number of ailments. Today, this bane of gardeners is appreciated most for its nutritional content. Dandelion greens are rich in beta-carotene and vitamin C and contain good amounts of B vitamins, calcium, iron, potassium, magnesium, and zinc as well. Dandelion root has a slight laxative effect; the greens act as a mild diuretic. Traditionally, dandelion has been prescribed by herbalists to treat diabetes, liver disease, and anemia. However, there is no reason to think that dandelion has any positive effect at all on these conditions.

❖ Deadly Nightshade

Atropa belladonna

Although deadly nightshade is the source of many valuable medicines, including atropine, hyoscyamine, and scopolamine, all parts of the plant are extremely poisonous. Never attempt to make any sort of herbal remedy from deadly nightshade.

❖ Devil's Claw

Harpagophytum procumbens

Because a German study in 1976 claimed that devil's claw, the root of a South African plant, had significant value as an anti-inflammatory for treating the pain and stiffness of arthritis, this herb had been touted as something of a wonder drug by natural medicine practitioners. Later studies failed to confirm the original finding, however. At this point, the only thing wondrous about devil's claw is the price. It is far more expensive than the drugs routinely prescribed for arthritis.

❖ Dill

Anethum graveolens

A member of the same plant family as carrot, celery, and parsley, dill has feathery leaves and a flat crown of tiny yellow flowers. Dill has always been a valuable commodity. In ancient Rome, heroic warriors were rewarded with crowns of dill flowers. The ancient Egyptians recognized its sooth-

ing effects on the digestive tract, while the Greeks believed
it cured hiccups. During the Middle Ages, people believed
that hanging dill above a door or carrying it with them
would keep them safe against evil spells and witchcraft.

Both dill seed and leaves are used in herbal medicine. The
name comes from the Saxon word *dilla,* which means to
lull, and dill has been traditionally used as a mild sedative
and a calming agent for the digestive tract. Tea made from
dill seed is said to help relieve gas pain and stomach upsets;
it is also said to help insomnia. Traditionally, dill tea is recommended to nursing mothers to increase their flow of milk.
Chewing on dill seeds is a pleasant remedy for bad breath.

One of the most common culinary uses of dill is as a pick-
ling spice and preservative. It is also widely used in many
Scandinavian dishes, and you will find it to be a great addition to your herbal repertoire. Fresh dill, which is definitely
preferable to dried dill, is often available in the produce section at the supermarket or from greengrocers. It is also easy
to grow in a sunny spot in the garden or on a windowsill.
The feathery leaves are best if used before the heads flower.
Dried dill and dill seed can be purchased in the spice section. The seeds and leaves have a similar flavor, although
the seeds are much stronger. Add dill near the end of the
cooking process to retain the most flavor. Because dill is
rich in mineral salts, it's a great flavoring for people on a
salt-free diet.

❖ Dock

See Yellow Dock.

❖ Dong Quai

Angelica sinensis

In traditional Chinese herbal medicine, dong quai (also known as dang gui) is used as a remedy for gynecological complaints. For that reason, it's sometimes called female ginseng. Chinese herbal practitioners prescribe it for premenstrual syndrome, menstrual cramps, and for regulating the menstrual cycle. It's also sometimes recommended for high blood pressure and treating anemia.

Dong quai does contain numerous coumarins, chemical compounds that have various effects, including relaxing blood vessels and relieving muscle spasms. However, dong quai also contains psoralens and other furocoumarins, chemical compounds that can cause, among other things, photosensitivity and dermatitis. In general, there is only anecdotal evidence to show that dong quai is effective, and the large amounts of furocoumarins in dong quai make it unacceptable as an herbal remedy.

See also Angelica.

❖ Echinacea

Echinacea angustifolia and *E. purpurea*

Commonly known as purple coneflower, echinacea was considered an essential healing herb by the Native Americans of the central plains. Its roots were used to treat toothaches, snakebite, fevers, wounds, and insect bites. Echinacea was embraced by the early settlers as a general cure-all, and it was widely used in many patent remedies in the nineteenth and early twentieth centuries. Once antibiotics such as sulfa became widely available in the 1930s, echinacea's popularity declined. In recent years, however, there has been a resurgence of interest in echinacea. A popular herbal remedy, it is also now the subject of a considerable number of scientific studies.

Echinacea root itself is not an antibiotic. As recent research has shown, its beneficial value comes from the stimulating effect it has on the immune system. Echinacea extracts taken orally can help increase your production of infection-fighting cells and boost their effectiveness. This in turn can help you fight off infections. In particular, echinacea does seem to really help some people ward off common colds or get over them faster. In conjunction with standard antibiotic treatment, echinacea may also help prevent the recurrence of respiratory and urinary tract infections or reduce their severity.

On the other hand, some claims for echinacea are exaggerated. Although it may have some value for helping to prevent infection in people with AIDS, it is not a substitute for medical treatment. Furthermore, proponents of echinacea claim that it can restore normal immune function in radiation patients and fight off influenza, herpes, and yeast infections. However, there is no real evidence that echinacea has a beneficial effect on these conditions, nor is there any evidence to suggest it helps arthritis, psoriasis, or such chronic illnesses as multiple sclerosis.

The usual dose of echinacea is 15 to 30 drops of an alcohol-based extract two to five times daily. Tea made from echinacea and capsules containing powdered echinacea root are not recommended, since some of the active ingredients are not water soluble. Some herbalists believe that the benefits of echinacea rise for four days and then drop off, and therefore recommend a regimen of four days on and four days off. Echinacea is easily confused with a plant known as prairie dock or Missouri snakeroot. Purchase your echinacea extract only from a reliable manufacturer.

❖ Elderberry

Sambucus spp.

Elderberry has a long and varied history. Believed to possess magical properties during the Middle Ages, it was made into a cosmetic to whiten skin in the eighteenth century, and was used as a healing herb by the Shakers. However, elderberry must be used with great caution because the leaves, bark, and roots have cyanide-containing compounds in them. Do not use these parts of the bush for any purpose. When cooked, the bush's ripe berries may be used harmlessly in jam. Elderberry flowers make a mild tea that some herbalists say acts as a mild stimulant. Although no real evidence supports this claim, in moderate amounts elder flower tea is a pleasant and enjoyable drink that does contain some vitamin A and vitamin C.

❖ Elecampane

Inula helenium

Elecampane has been used medicinally as far back as ancient Greece and Rome to treat respiratory problems, and herbalists today still recommend it for the same purpose. Traditionally used to treat coughs and other minor respiratory ailments, elecampane tea helps clear up bronchial congestion and has a soothing effect on the respiratory tract. To make elecampane tea, steep 3 tablespoons of crushed root in 2 cups of boiling water for fifteen minutes. Let cool and strain. Stir in 2 tablespoons of honey. Drink 1/2 cup every three hours.

Elecampane also has a mild diuretic effect and is said to help relieve mild menstrual cramps, stomach cramps, and indigestion.

❖ Eleuthero
See Siberian Ginseng.

❖ Ephedra

***Ephedra* spp.**

Ephedra, also known by its Chinese name ma huang, has traditionally been used as an asthma medication in China and India for thousands of years. This herb can be an effective remedy in mild cases because ephedra contains ephedrine and other related alkaloids that relieve bronchial spasm and stimulate the central nervous system. In synthetic form, ephedrine is found in some prescription asthma medications and in many over-the-counter cold and allergy remedies. In addition to helping to relieve mild asthma symptoms, ephedra is an effective decongestant that can relieve cold and allergy symptoms, such as stuffy nose, watery eyes, and cough.

For relieving congestion and coughing, herbalists generally recommend drinking a tea made from 1 heaping teaspoon ephedra steeped in 16 ounces of boiling water for ten minutes. If an asthma attack is imminent or already under way, never substitute ephedra for the medication prescribed by your doctor. The herb takes too long to act. Stop using ephedra or use less of it if it causes nervousness, headaches, dizziness, or insomnia.

Because ephedrine is a stimulant that increases your body's basal metabolic rate, ephedra is sometimes combined with other herbs such as uva ursi in weight-loss teas. Using ephedra to lose weight could lead to insomnia, irritability, and other potentially serious problems, however, and it is definitely not recommended.

Ephedra's stimulating effects are so strong that it is on the U.S. Olympic Committee's list of banned substances. Do not use ephedra if you have high blood pressure, glaucoma, heart disease, diabetes, an overactive thyroid, or any other chronic condition. Avoid ephedra during pregnancy or if you suffer from insomnia. If you have asthma or emphysema, discuss taking ephedra with your doctor before you try it.

Mormon tea, a North American herb also called squaw tea, desert herb, or Brigham Young weed, is a species of ephedra, but it does not contain any of the alkaloid substances found in the Chinese species, and it has no effect on asthma or hay fever.

❖ Eucalyptus

Eucalyptus spp.

A tall tree with silvery leaves, the eucalyptus is native to Australia. Its leaves are the chief food of the koala bear, and they contain a strongly aromatic oil. Eucalyptus oil is highly effective for relieving cold symptoms such as stuffy sinuses and clogged bronchial tubes. It's a common ingredient in over-the-counter cough drops, throat lozenges, and nasal sprays. You can also make your own eucalyptus decongestant by boiling 6 leaves in 1 quart of water for twenty minutes. Add the water to your vaporizer; alternatively, use plain water in the vaporizer and add a few drops of eucalyptus oil.

Eucalyptus also increases the blood flow when it is rubbed on the skin. The warm feeling this produces can help to ease sore muscles and relieve the stiffness and pain of arthritis. However, undiluted eucalyptus oil can be very irritating to the skin and should be avoided. Instead, try a liniment or cream that contains eucalyptus oil.

Some herbalists recommend diluted eucalyptus oil as a treatment for dandruff and minor skin irritations. It can also be used as an antiseptic for minor cuts and scrapes. A word of caution: Do not use eucalyptus oil in or near the eyes, mouth, nose, or genitals. More than a couple of drops of eucalyptus oil taken internally can be toxic, so it is best to avoid ingesting any preparations that contain it.

Eucalyptus oil has another valuable use as an insect repellent. Rub diluted eucalyptus oil on your skin to keep mosquitoes away. A piece of cloth soaked in eucalyptus oil may help repel cockroaches.

❖ Evening Primrose Oil

Oenothera biennis

So named because the flowers of this aromatic plant, a native of North America, open at dusk, oil from its seeds was traditionally used by the Native Americans as a sedative and painkiller. Today, the oil is the subject of ongoing scientific study because it contains large amounts of essential fatty acid gamma-linolenic acid (GLA), a type of fat your body can't manufacture on its own. GLA is used by your body to make prostaglandins, powerful hormonelike substances necessary for regulating a number of body functions.

Natural medicine practitioners and herbalists make numerous broad claims for evening primrose oil. It is said to lower blood cholesterol levels and reduce high blood pressure. Many women say that evening primrose oil capsules relieve PMS symptoms such as headache, bloating, and breast tenderness. Evening primrose oil is sometimes recommended as a treatment for eczema, multiple sclerosis, diabetes, and arthritis. It has even been reputed to cure hangovers and allow you to lose weight while you sleep.

As with any remedy that is said to be a cure-all for a wide range of ailments, the claims for evening primrose oil must be viewed with great skepticism. Although some studies have shown positive results, other studies have not, and still others have contradicted the results of earlier studies. To date, there is no real evidence that GLA has a substantial beneficial effect on any of the problems mentioned above or on any other condition. If you wish to try evening primrose oil to treat a chronic condition, discuss it with your doctor first.

Evening primrose oil capsules are readily available at any health food store. They are expensive, and since they are easy to dilute with cheaper soy or safflower oil, be sure you are purchasing a good product from a reputable manufacturer.

See also Borage.

❖ Eyebright

Euphrasia officinalis

Eyebright is a traditional remedy for eye ailments, despite the lack of any evidence to prove it does any good. For itchy, red, burning, or bloodshot eyes, herbal medicine practitioners sometimes suggest swallowing eyebright capsules or drinking eyebright tea. More commonly, and unwisely, they recommend using eyebright as an eyewash. However, putting anything that isn't sterile into your eyes is dangerous. Herbal eyewashes won't help your irritated eyes and they could cause an infection. Do not use any sort of herbal eyewash, homemade or purchased.

A cool compress made from a clean washcloth soaked in cold water can help soothe red, tired eyes. Lie down, place the compress on your closed eyes, and rest for ten minutes; repeat if necessary.

If you wish to use eyebright capsules or tea, be certain that you are buying European eyebright *(Euphrasia)* and not any other herb.

❖ Fennel

Foeniculum vulgare

With its feathery cap of leaves and celerylike stalks, fennel looks a lot like dill, but it tastes more like anise or licorice. The stalks are an excellent dietary source of vitamin A and potassium.

Tea made from fennel seeds is traditionally recommended for promoting milk in breast-feeding mothers (although it is probably the extra liquid, not the fennel itself, that helps). Fennel seed tea can help settle an upset stomach and relieve indigestion and a few drops added to the bottle can often calm a colicky baby. Chewing on fennel seeds can freshen your breath. However, avoid fennel seed oil—it is quite volatile and can be irritating to the skin.

❖ Fenugreek

Trigonella foenumgraecum

Fenugreek is one of the oldest medicinal herbs. In ancient Greece, it was added to the feed of sick animals to encourage them to eat. In ancient Egypt, it was used to ease childbirth and increase milk flow. In ancient India, it was used to treat arthritis and bronchitis, and in ancient China, it was used to treat fevers. During the nineteenth century, fenugreek was a popular ingredient in many American patent medicines.

Although fenugreek is no longer considered a cure-all, it still has some value as an herbal remedy. Fenugreek seeds contain a relatively high level of mucilage, which makes them valuable as a natural laxative and as an aid to such minor digestive problems as heartburn. Fenugreek tea is traditionally recommended for indigestion, coughs, and menstrual cramps. Warm fenugreek tea may also be used as a gargle to give some relief from a sore throat. Externally, a poultice or ointment of crushed fenugreek seeds is sometimes recommended by herbalists to relieve minor skin inflammations and rashes.

Fenugreek is traditionally used as a treatment for diabetes in Indian and Chinese herbal medicine. Some recent animal studies suggest that it may indeed have some beneficial effect on diabetes and on high blood cholesterol as well, but there is no evidence pertaining to humans. If you have diabetes, high blood cholesterol, or any other condition you'd like to treat with fenugreek, speak to your doctor first.

❖ Feverfew

Chrysanthemum parthenium

Feverfew has been used as an herbal treatment for a wide range of ailments, particularly fevers, as its common name suggests, but for most purposes it has little or no medicinal value. Feverfew is under active investigation, however, for the treatment of migraine headaches. Studies have shown that feverfew leaves contain a substance that relaxes the blood vessels in the brain. Patients who eat a few fresh feverfew leaves or take feverfew capsules or extract every day have fewer and less severe migraines, although the treatment may take several months to become effective. You can buy feverfew capsules and extracts at health food stores, but be aware that many of these products contain little of the active ingredient in feverfew. Although this herb shows promise as a migraine treatment, you should discuss it with your doctor before trying it. Feverfew can affect your blood clotting rates and can interfere with certain prescription drugs.

❖ Fish Oil

Omega-3 fatty acid, or fish oil, is used by your body to make eicosapentanoic acid (EPA), which in turn is needed to make hormonelike substances called prostaglandins. Among other things, protaglandins help discourage heart disease by keeping your blood flowing normally, preventing the buildup of plaque in your arteries, and reducing the chances of dangerous blood clots. Fish oil can raise your HDL (good) cholesterol and lower your triglyceride levels; it can also help lower your blood pressure.

According to the National Heart and Lung Institute, a single gram of omega-3 fatty acids daily (about the amount in a 3-ounce serving of fish) could reduce the risk of cardiovascular disease in men. Just how substantial the reduction might be is somewhat controversial. A recent study of American men who routinely ate fish two or three times a week showed no reduction in their rate of cardiovascular disease, even when other factors such as cigarette smoking and exercise were taken into account. In short, there's no guarantee that fish oil will keep you from having a heart attack.

Fish oil is also recommended by natural medicine practitioners as a treatment for menstrual discomfort, PMS symptoms, migraine headaches, psoriasis, eczema, arthritis, and other problems. While one or two fish oil capsules a day are unlikely to hurt you, there is little evidence that they will help. If you have diabetes, do not use fish oil capsules, as they can cause your blood sugar level to rise.

❖ Flaxseed

Linum usitatissimum

Also known as linseed, flaxseed has a high mucilage content, which makes it a good natural bulking remedy for constipation. To get the best effect, try adding 2 teaspoons of flaxseed to your breakfast cereal or swallow them mixed with honey. Drink one to two full glasses of liquid immediately after eating the seeds. Flaxseed is also rich in linoleic and linolenic acids.

Flaxseed oil, also known as linseed oil, is said to be a good concentrated source of essential fatty acids and is also sometimes recommended for coughs. However, linseed oil contains cyanidelike compounds and should not be used medicinally.

❖ Fo-Ti

Polygonum multiflorum

Also sometimes called he-shou-wu, fo-ti is used in traditional Chinese medicine as a rejuvenating tonic purported to relieve the signs and symptoms of aging. Although the belief that fo-ti can keep your hair from graying is completely unfounded, another use of fo-ti does have validity: It is an effective cathartic for the relief of constipation. Doctors generally advise against using cathartics, however, and therefore fo-ti should be avoided.

❖ Foxglove

Digitalis purpurea

Foxglove provided one of the earliest successful treatments for congestive heart failure back in the late 1700s, when the dried leaves of the purple foxglove plant were noted to contain digitalis. This powerful drug increases the force of your heart contractions. Since the 1940s, an even more powerful drug for heart failure, digoxin, has been made from foxglove. Foxglove is a popular garden flower, but it is extremely dangerous to treat congestive heart failure on your own with homemade digitalis. Many deaths have resulted from ingesting foxglove.

❖ Garlic

Allium sativum

A member of the lily family and related to the onion, garlic has been used to add flavor to other foods for over 5,000 years. However, its reputation in folk medicine is nothing short of remarkable: it has been credited as a laxative, diuretic, sedative, antiseptic, and as a remedy for a multitude of maladies including gastrointestinal disorders, animal bites, hemorrhoids, ulcers, loss of appetite, tumors, and heart disease. It even has been acclaimed as an aphrodisiac. In fact, the truth is pretty remarkable, too. Garlic contains numerous compounds that have shown evidence of helping to prevent heart disease, stroke, cancer, high cholesterol, and infections. To get the maximum protective effects of garlic, doctors recommend two or three cloves a day, raw or cooked.

Garlic as an Antibiotic

During both world wars, doctors were forced to improvise when medical supplies ran short. They discovered that garlic is a potent antibiotic that helped wounds heal. In Russia, garlic is known as Russian penicillin, and 500 tons were once rushed there to deal with an influenza outbreak. Allicin, the compound that releases its pungent odor when garlic is cut or crushed, was once thought to be responsible for garlic's benefits. Actually, it's the sulfur-containing compounds formed by the breakdown of allicin that give garlic its pharmacological effects.

Garlic as Heart Helper

By reducing your blood's clotting ability (lessening the stickiness of blood platelets), garlic helps prevent the formation of life-threatening blood clots. Garlic can also help improve blood cholesterol levels by lowering LDL (bad) cholesterol levels and raising HDL (good) cholesterol levels, and it can also help lower levels of the potentially harmful blood fats known as triglycerides.

Garlic as Anticancer Aid

Animal studies suggest that garlic can help protect against cancers caused by exposure to carcinogens. Other studies indicate that garlic may help prevent metastasis, or the spread of cancer cells from their original site to other parts of the body. Garlic contains some fifteen potent antioxidant substances that help fight cancer and other diseases.

Garlic as Blood Pressure Stabilizer

The Japanese government officially recognizes garlic as a blood pressure depressor. In laboratory animals, garlic consistently lowers blood pressure levels. Studies on humans have also shown a drop in systolic and diastolic blood pressure when garlic was consumed.

Garlic as Common Cold Fighter

Garlic seems to work the way most over-the-counter expectorants and decongestants do: it irritates the stomach, which signals to the lungs to release fluids that thin out mucus, and that helps your lungs expel it.

Using Garlic

To obtain optimal healing properties, don't swallow whole garlic cloves—chew, chop, or crush them. Eating garlic, although good for your health, can be hazardous to your breath. To help eliminate the odor, try chewing some fresh parsley sprigs or a few fennel seeds afterwards. It's impossible to completely eliminate garlic's aroma when taking medicinal quantities of it, however. Garlic supplements, such as Kyolic, are sold as liquids or as capsules containing dried garlic. If you don't like to eat garlic in your food, try taking the supplements instead. You can get the benefit without the odor.

Before you start using medicinal amounts of garlic, discuss it with your doctor. In some cases (clotting disorders, for instance), taking garlic would not be advised. Furthermore, some people have experienced toxic reactions when taking over ten raw cloves a day.

❖ Gentian

Gentiana lutea

Gentian root has long been used as an herbal aid to digestion. It is still used today as a digestive bitter in some liqueurs and as the ingredient that gives Angostura bitters its characteristic flavor. In America in the late 1800s, Beverage Moxie Nerve Food was hawked as a curative for a variety of ills, including impotence and nervous exhaustion. Though the bitter beverage never proved useful for boosting male potency or fortitude, Moxie caught on as a soft drink that is still sold today, and the word *moxie,* meaning courage or determination, was coined.

Gentian root is sometimes used today as an appetite and digestive stimulant. Modern herbalists often recommend it as a general tonic, but despite claims, there is nothing in gentian that can help arthritis, fevers, menstrual discomfort, gallstones, or liver disease.

❖ Ginger

Zingiber officinale

Native to Asia and cultivated in many tropical areas today, the ginger plant has a knotty, fibrous root that is widely used as a spice and herbal medicine. The pungent taste of ginger is used extensively in Asian cooking. It's also used in ginger ale, ginger snaps, and gingerbread and as a scent to perfume soaps, shampoos, and fragrances.

In traditional Asian medicine, ginger is widely used for nearly all medical problems. Ginger tea can help stimulate the appetite, relieve heartburn and flatulence, and help coughs. It is said to help reduce the swelling, pain, and stiffness of arthritis and aid the circulatory system, although there is no evidence to back this up. Neither is there any evidence to support claims that ginger can reduce high blood pressure, high cholesterol, or high blood sugar.

Ginger does have a valuable, well-documented use as a treatment for motion sickness. It seems to work best if taken about twenty minutes before the trip begins. The form of the ginger doesn't seem to matter much. Try swallowing 1/2 teaspoon of ground ginger (mixed in water or placed in a gelatin capsule), eating a small piece of fresh gingerroot, having a cup of gingerroot tea, or eating a few pieces of candied ginger. Don't overdo it, however. Too much ginger can cause mouth and intestinal irritation. You can buy fresh and dried gingerroot at supermarkets and greengrocers. Pickled ginger can be purchased at Asian grocery stores, and ginger capsules are available at health food stores and some pharmacies. Consumers should be aware that the ground ginger that is available as a spice is not the same as the dried ginger used in traditional Chinese medicine.

❖ Ginkgo

Ginkgo biloba

When the ginkgo tree was brought to Europe from China in the 1700s, its purpose was purely ornamental, even though the Chinese prized the leaves for their medicinal value. More than two hundred years later, Western medicine has discovered the same. Over the past few decades, ginkgo biloba extract (GBE) has been carefully studied for its ability to relax and dilate blood vessels. GBE can be a helpful treatment for promoting blood flow to the brain, heart, and lower extremities, particularly for elderly patients, which is good news for those who suffer from ailments related to narrowed arteries. GBE can be taken as a preventive for people at risk of stroke, and after a stroke, it can speed recovery. Among the elderly, ginkgo can increase blood flow to the brain and help short-term memory loss. It may have some value for Alzheimer's disease, particularly when taken in fluid extract form. Ginkgo in liquid, capsule, or tablet form could also help relieve varicose veins, tinnitus, and Raynaud's disease symptoms.

Ginkgo leaf extract is widely prescribed by German doctors and is also available in Germany in over-the-counter preparations. In the United States, GBE is sold chiefly in health food stores. Consumers are advised to purchase GBE only from a reputable manufacturer. Don't take ginkgo biloba if you are taking any sort of blood-thinning medication or if you have a blood clotting disorder. If you wish to try ginkgo biloba for any medical problem, discuss it with your doctor first. Very large doses of GBE could cause nausea, diarrhea, and other side effects.

❖ Ginseng

Panax ginseng

The ginseng root has been valued in traditional Chinese herbal medicine for over five thousand years. In addition to being recommended for almost every ailment that exists, it is also said to promote long life, decrease the effects of aging, and act as an aphrodisiac. While most of the claims made for ginseng are wildly exaggerated or based purely on superstition, ginseng does have some value as an herbal medicine. Its chief value seems to be as an adaptogen, a substance that helps normalize body functions and helps you cope better with both physical and emotional stress. Many people claim that drinking ginseng tea helps them recover more quickly from minor illnesses such as colds or flu. Ginseng can also act as a mild stimulant that boosts energy, increases endurance, and counteracts fatigue, but it can also cause insomnia in some people. It is often recommended as a tonic to strengthen the body for winter weather. Sadly, there is no evidence that it is an aphrodisiac.

Two types of real ginseng are sold in health food stores and Oriental specialty stores: Chinese or Korean ginseng and American ginseng. (Siberian ginseng is a completely different herb.) A great deal of confusion exists as to which exactly is the genuine ginseng root. The active ingredients— triterpenoid saponins—are identical in both, but herbalists claim that the wild American root is superior for "cold" conditions such as lung problems. The finest ginseng is said to come from Korea, with wild American ginseng not far behind. Purchase your ginseng only from a reliable supplier. It is easy to adulterate or fake. In addition, many herbal mixtures and teas said to contain ginseng as an ingredient in fact have virtually none.

Ginseng is usually taken as a tea made from the powdered root. To prepare ginseng tea, steep 1 to 3 teaspoonfuls of ginseng in 1 cup boiling water for ten minutes, stirring occasionally. Stir before drinking. Ginseng tablets and capsules are available in various dosages. Herbalists generally suggest daily doses ranging from 500 milligrams to 2 grams.

Avoid ginseng if you have insomnia, high blood pressure, a clotting disorder, or are pregnant. Stop taking it if you develop nausea, diarrhea, or skin eruptions.

See also Canaigre; Siberian Ginseng.

❖ Goldenrod

Solidago spp.

It's hard to believe that a weed so reviled by hay fever sufferers could have any value, but in fact, goldenrod is a useful herb for treating kidney stones because it is a diuretic, and an increased urine flow can help you pass a kidney stone. For the same reason, goldenrod is sometimes used to treat the symptoms of urinary tract infections. To make goldenrod tea, steep 2 teaspoons of the flowers in 2 cups of boiling water. Let stand for twenty minutes, strain, and drink.

Goldenrod, sometimes mixed with uva ursi (bearberry), is often recommended as a weight-loss tea. Drinking this mixture will lead to some immediate water weight loss due to increased urination, but the loss will be only temporary. Do not use diuretic herbs for weight loss.

❖ Goldenseal

Hydrastis canadensis

Once used by Native Americans, goldenseal root today is still recommended for a wide range of uses. For an herb this popular and expensive, it does surprisingly little.

Goldenseal root is purported to have antibiotic and antifungal properties and is also said to boost the immune system by stimulating the production of white blood cells. Many volumes on herbal lore have variously recommended goldenseal as a treatment for yeast infections, as an antiseptic for wounds, as a mouthwash for preventing gum disease and treating mouth sores, as a mild laxative, and as treatments for conjunctivitis, eczema, hemorrhoids, ringworm, athlete's foot, gastritis, diarrhea, and even amoebic dysentery and cholera. Obviously, no herb could possibly treat all of these medical problems. Goldenseal's medicinal value is negligible. It does contain hydrastine, a compound that can act as a mild stimulant on the central nervous system, and it does have some minor effect on the circulatory system. It also has some mild antibiotic activity and is somewhat effective as an astringent and antiseptic for relieving mouth irritation. In general, however, the doses needed to achieve these effects are quite large and potentially toxic. In addition, since hydrastine can accumulate in your body's tissues, even taking small doses of goldenseal could eventually have a toxic effect. Avoid this herb.

❖ Gotu Kola

Centella asiatica

Legend in Sri Lanka has it that eating two leaves of gotu kola a day will vastly increase your longevity. This popular Indian herb is said to improve the immune system and accelerate the healing of wounds and burns. It is also said to be helpful as a sedative and painkiller. In addition, gotu kola has a reputation as an aphrodisiac.

Animal studies show that gotu kola contains glycerides that do have a sedative effect and may have some value for stimulating wound healing and relieving inflammation. However, gotu kola is not an aphrodisiac. This herb has not been thoroughly researched. Use it with caution if at all.

❖ Hawthorn

Crataegus oxyacantha

Also known as mayflower, hawthorn is a small to medium-sized shrubby tree native to Europe. Traditionally, herbal remedies based on hawthorn leaves, flowers, and berries have been recommended in Europe for treating heart disease—a use modern research is confirming. Bioflavonoids in hawthorn can help dilate blood vessels, lower blood pressure, and help damaged hearts repair themselves. In Germany, hawthorn preparations are regularly prescribed for minor heart conditions. The effects of hawthorn on the heart develop slowly and cumulatively. It should be used only as a supplemental tonic, not as a primary treatment for a heart condition or as a substitute for any drugs your doctor prescribes. Discuss using hawthorn with your doctor before you try it.

Hawthorn is also a mild sedative that can be very good for stress and nervous conditions, as well as insomnia. To treat these, take 1 cup of hawthorn tea two or three times daily.

❖ Honey

Because honey is a natural product made by bees from flower nectar, some people believe it is somehow better for you than refined table sugar. In fact, honey is made mostly of sucrose, exactly the same substance as table sugar (although honey also contains fructose and glucose). If you should avoid sweeteners such as sugar (if you have diabetes, for example), you should also avoid honey. Furthermore, a tablespoon of honey contains about 64 calories, roughly 20 more calories than an equivalent amount of table sugar.

Because honey contains antimicrobial substances, it has been used for centuries to treat wounds and burns. (Never try to treat severe or infected wounds and burns with honey. See your doctor instead.) A traditional remedy for coughs and sore throats is a syrup made of honey and garlic.

❖ Honeysuckle

Lonicera spp.

Honeysuckle, also known as woodbine, is a twining shrub with fragrant yellow or white flowers. Native to Asia, it now grows wild in North America, particularly in the northeastern United States. Tea made from honeysuckle flowers has a soothing effect on upper respiratory irritations due to colds, coughs, sore throats, bronchitis, and laryngitis. A syrup made from the flowers is a traditional European cough remedy. Use only the flowers because honeysuckle berries are toxic.

❖ Hops

Humulus lupulus

The cone-shaped, scaly fruits of the hop plant have been used to flavor and preserve beer since the ninth century. Also used as a digestive bitter for centuries, hops are primarily used in herbal medicine as a sedative. Pillows filled with hops (sometimes mixed with lavender for a more pleasant aroma) are a traditional remedy for insomnia and bad dreams. Tea made from hops is recommended for nervousness, mild anxiety, insomnia, and stress. Try 1 cup of hops tea three times a day for a mild tranquilizing effect. Hops tea is also suggested by herbalists for calming upset stomachs. Their mild antiseptic action also can make them useful in a poultice for minor skin irritations.

Fresh hops are the most effective; the fruits lose much of their potency when stored.

❖ Horehound

Marrubium vulgare

Horehound, a member of the mint family, has been used to treat coughs and sore throats for centuries. The leaves and flowering tops of this plant have a strong, characteristic taste that is used today as a flavoring in many commercial throat lozenges, cough drops, and cough syrups. (The FDA does not recognize horehound as a drug.)

Horehound can be a useful home remedy for sore throats and coughs; it also has some value as an expectorant. Steep 1 teaspoon of horehound leaves in 1 cup of boiling water. Take 1 tablespoon every three hours. Do not take more than 1 cup daily.

Horseradish

Armoracia rusticana

A pungent root vegetable related to mustard, horseradish was once used to alleviate asthma and treat kidney diseases. Although used primarily in the kitchen as a pungent condiment, horseradish still has some value as a decongestant for relieving cold, flu, and sinusitis symptoms. An old folk remedy for stuffy noses, sore throats, and coughs is a hot mixture of honey, freshly grated horseradish, and hot water. Do not take large quantities at one time as diarrhea could result.

❖ Horsetail

Equisetum spp.

The last of an almost extinct family, horsetail is a descendant of the plants that covered the earth 200 million years ago. This rushlike plant has hollow stems, scalelike leaves, and reproduces by spores. In traditional herbal medicine, horsetail has been used to heal wounds and stop bleeding; it was also recommended for bladder and urinary tract problems as well as a range of other ailments, including stomach ulcers and tuberculosis. Modern research reveals that horsetail does have a weak diuretic effect. The broader claims made for it by herbalists are unfounded. In fact, horsetail in large quantities can be toxic, so this is an herb to avoid.

❖ Hyssop

Hyssopus officinalis

Hyssop, a hardy, perennial shrub, grows in sun or light shade with very little care, and it is great for attracting bees, butterflies, and hummingbirds into your garden. Hyssop is a member of the mint family and has a strong, camphorlike aroma (familiar to some as an ingredient in the liqueurs Benedictine and Chartreuse). It may even have some worthwhile medicinal qualities. Taken as a tea or a gargle, it is a moderately useful home remedy for treating mild upper respiratory problems due to colds, coughs, and flu. Use the leaves and flowering tops to make a tea. Take no more than 2 cups a day. For a more enjoyable flavor, try combining equal parts hyssop and horehound.

Some herbalists say that hyssop is an antibiotic and antiseptic for wounds, particularly puncture wounds or those made by rusty metal. This claim seems to be based on the fact that penicillin mold grows on hyssop leaves. This is fractured science, however. Penicillin mold grows on lots of things (just open the vegetable bin or bread box after a long vacation), but that does not make them antibiotics. Do not use hyssop leaves to treat any sort of wound.

❖ Iceland Moss

Cetraria islandica

Iceland moss is actually a lichen found in Scandinavia and central Europe. It has a high mucilage content that makes it a soothing treatment for upper respiratory irritation; it is also a useful herbal cough remedy. The usual dose is 3 to 4 teaspoons of dried Iceland moss steeped in 1 cup of boiling water. Take no more than 1 cup three times a day. Because Iceland moss contains some lead, do not use it for more than a few days, and don't give it to children.

❖ Ipecac

Cephaelis ipecacuanha or *C. acuminata*

Ipecac, a root from South America, has two medicinal uses: as an emetic and as an expectorant. Nonprescription ipecac syrup is sold in pharmacies as an emetic used to induce vomiting in cases of poisoning. As an ingredient in prescription and nonprescription cough syrups, ipecac can be helpful as an expectorant for coughs. In either case, read labels carefully and use only as directed. Do not attempt to make home remedies from ipecac.

❖ Irish Moss

Chondius crispus

Irish moss is actually seaweed found along the Atlantic coasts of Europe. It has a high mucilage content that can be useful for relieving upper respiratory irritation and coughs when taken as a tea. Applied externally as a poultice, it is sometimes helpful for relieving minor skin irritations and rashes.

❖ Jasmine

Jasminum officinale

The fragrant blossoms of jasmine have been brewed into a relaxing tea for centuries. Try adding some jasmine flowers to your bathwater for a serene time-out. Some people believe that jasmine oil acts as an aphrodisiac when rubbed on the body, but that's a subjective evaluation you'll have to determine for yourself.

❖ Jimsonweed

Datura stramonium
Jimsonweed has been used over the centuries, including in recent times, as a hallucinogen. Also known as datura, thorn apple, and loco weed, among other colorful descriptions, jimsonweed grows wild by the roadside in most parts of North America. Its flowers resemble those of morning glory. However, do not use jimsonweed in any form or for any reason. This plant is highly toxic. Even touching it can cause skin irritation. Ingesting or smoking jimsonweed can cause serious illness or even death.

❖ Jojoba Oil

Simmondsia chinensis or *S. californica*
An evergreen shrub that grows in the rocky desert regions of the American Southwest, jojoba (pronounced ho-HO-ba) produces numerous beanlike seeds. When crushed, the seeds contain an abundance of a waxy substance commonly called jojoba oil. Proponents of jojoba say it cures everything from baldness to cancer, but of course there is no substantiation to these wild claims. What is true about jojoba is that it is very effective as a lotion for dry skin and as a conditioner for the

hair. Accordingly, jojoba oil is often incorporated into commercial skin creams and hair conditioners.

❖ Juniper Berries

Juniperus communis

In the sixteenth century, a Dutch pharmacist soaked the berries of the evergreen juniper shrub in distilled alcohol and offered it to the public as a new drug. English-speaking people called it gin (after the Dutch word for juniper, *genever*) and, like their Continental counterparts, drank it for pleasure. While gin is far from medicinal, juniper berries do have some healing value. In particular, the berries are an effective diuretic (but only if fresh berries are used). Traditionally, tea made from juniper berries was recommended by herbalists to treat kidney and bladder problems. This can irritate the kidneys, however, and should be avoided by people with kidney disease. Juniper can also cause uterine contractions and should not be taken by pregnant women. In general, if a diuretic is needed, safer choices are available.

❖ Kelp
See Seaweed.

❖ Kola

Cola acuminata

The kola tree, native to West Africa and now cultivated in South America and the West Indies, bears a nutlike seed that contains caffeine. Because the kola nut was traditionally said to have generic medicinal qualities, in the late 1800s a pharmacist mixed a syrup of kola, coca (the source of cocaine), and sugar with carbonated water. He created not a medicine but the basic formula for Coca-Cola. Although the narcotic coca is no longer an ingredient, Coke still contains kola as a primary flavoring ingredient. Despite traditional claims, however, there is no real use for kola nuts in herbal medicine today.

❖ Kombu
See Seaweed.

Lady's Mantle

Alchemilla vulgaris

Lady's mantle gets its name from the scalloped edges of its leaves, which resemble the cloak of the Virgin Mary in medieval paintings. Perhaps because of its association with the Virgin, lady's mantle has a reputation as an herb for "women's troubles."

Lady's mantle is often suggested specifically for heavy menstrual bleeding and for relieving vaginal itching; it is sometimes used as a general tonic for menopausal women. Does it work? For cramps due to heavy menstrual bleeding, probably no better than any other mild herbal tea. (If your menstrual bleeding is unusually heavy, see your doctor as soon as possible.) Used as an ointment, lady's mantle may temporarily help stop vaginal itching, but it will not affect the underlying problem. Speak to your doctor about treatment. As a general tonic for menopause, lady's mantle is probably worthless. Avoid lady's mantle if you are pregnant—this herb can be a uterine stimulant.

This astringent herb does have a high tannin content. Taken internally as a tea, it is helpful for relieving diarrhea. Used as a gargle, the cooled tea helps relieve discomfort from mouth sores and sore throat.

❖ Lavender

Lavandula angustifolia

Once a very popular healing herb, lavender is now used primarily for its delightful aroma in soaps, perfumes, sachets, and bath oils. But to use lavender only for its smell is to miss some of its healthful properties.

Lavender flowers are used in a traditional herbal tea for nerves. It does have a mildly sedative effect that can help relieve tension headaches and insomnia. Lavender oil—for external use only—is the more common form of this herb, however. Some migraine sufferers find they can fend off an attack if they lie down in a dark, quiet place at the first hint of a headache and rub a few drops of lavender oil into each temple. A drop or two of lavender oil rubbed into the affected area provides relief for insect bites and minor skin irritations. If you have a sunburn, try soaking in a tub of cool water with a few drops of lavender oil added.

❖ Lemon Balm
See Balm.

❖ Licorice

Glycyrrhiza glabra

Most of the licorice root imported to the United States is used to flavor tobacco products. This extremely unhealthy use of the root should not take away from its genuine medicinal value. Licorice root can be a useful treatment for peptic (stomach) ulcers. It is usually taken as a tea made from 1 teaspoonful of the licorice root steeped in 1/2 cup of water for five minutes. Strain before drinking; take 1/2 cup three times a day after meals.

Another valuable use of licorice root is as a cough medicine, either by itself or in combination with other herbal cough relievers such as horehound. Licorice is often used as an ingredient in nonprescription cough medicines and cough drops. Since many licorice-flavored products are actually flavored with anise, you should read the label carefully.

Licorice root can cause you to retain fluids. Don't use it if you have high blood pressure, heart disease, liver disease, or are pregnant. Stop using licorice root if you notice any swelling in your face, hands, or feet, and don't use it for longer than four weeks.

❖ Life Root

Senecia aureus

In the nineteenth century, life root was widely recommended for such "women's troubles" as irregular menstruation. Also called squaw weed, ragwort, and false valerian, it was an ingredient in many patent medicines marketed to women. Today, scientists know that life root contains dangerous alkaloids that can cause liver cancer. Do not use life root for any purpose.

❖ Linden Flowers

Tilia cordata* or *T. platyphyllos

The fragrant white or yellow flowers of the linden tree (also called basswood or lime tree) are used to make an aromatic, relaxing tea. In medieval times, linden was thought to be a useful treatment for ailments ranging from diarrhea to epilepsy, but today its only medicinal use is as a diaphoretic (a substance that induces sweating). To get the diaphoretic effect, however, you would have to drink quite a bit of tea. Since there is only rarely any medical reason to promote sweating, enjoy linden tea as a refreshing beverage.

❖ Lobelia

Lobelia inflata

Also called Indian tobacco, lobelia is a dangerous herb that should never be used internally, as even a small amount can cause vomiting, convulsions, and death. Because the effects of lobelia are somewhat similar to those of nicotine, lobelia is found in some over-the-counter products that allegedly help you stop smoking. Sold as tablets, lozenges, or chewing gum, these products claim to ease nicotine withdrawal symptoms, making it easier to quit smoking. Potentially dangerous, they have not been shown to be effective and should be avoided.

❖ Lovage

Levisticum officinale
The leaves of the lovage plant are often used as a seasoning for soups and stews. Lovage is also the principal flavor in Maggi sauce, a commercial seasoning liquid. The root of the lovage plant is the part that interests herbalists, however. Its primary use is as a diuretic, and it is often listed as an ingredient in weight-loss teas. Lovage root is effective for this purpose, but dieters should be aware that weight loss from diuretics is temporary, and overuse of diuretics is dangerous.

Lovage tea is also useful as a soothing drink to calm an upset stomach and relieve gas.

Frequent use of lovage can make your skin sensitive to light and could cause dermatitis.

❖ Ma Huang
See Ephedra.

❖ Marshmallow

Althaea officinalis

At one time the mucilage in marshmallow root was used to hold together a sugary white confection. Today's campfire marshmallows aren't made with the root, but the herb's high mucilage content makes it valuable as a home remedy for coughs and sore throats.

Marshmallow tea suppresses coughing and soothes sore throats. The dried root can be found in health food stores; marshmallow leaves and flowers are equally effective but can be hard to find. To make the tea, steep 2 teaspoons of chopped marshmallow roots, leaves, or flowers in 1 cup boiling water. Strain before using. Take 3 to 4 tablespoons every few hours, and take no more than one cup a day.

❖ Maté

Ilex paraguariensis

An extremely popular drink in South America, maté is made from the dried leaves of a type of holly found in southern Brazil, Argentina, and Paraguay. Also called yerba maté, yerba, or Paraguay tea, maté contains caffeine, although less than what is found in an equal amount of coffee or tea. Maté is a mild stimulant that can help relieve headaches, but it's mainly enjoyed as a refreshing beverage.

❖ Mayapple

Podophyllum peltatum
Found in moist woodland areas, mayapple, also sometimes called American mandrake or Indian apple, is a low-growing plant with large leaves. A single flower forms below the leaves of each plant; later, a fruit forms. Mayapple at one time was used as an herbal medicine and laxative, but the Food and Drug Administration lists it as unsafe. Mayapple is dangerously poisonous. Do not use it for any purpose.

❖ Meadowsweet

Filipendula ulmaria
For centuries in Europe, meadowsweet was traditionally recommended as an herbal remedy for the aches and pains of arthritis. Research in the nineteenth century revealed that meadowsweet contains salicylates, the same substance that is in aspirin. In fact, when acetylsalicylate was first synthesized in the 1890s, it was called aspirin after the old botanical name for meadowsweet, *Spirea*.

Today, the effects of meadowsweet can be achieved more quickly and to a greater degree by an aspirin tablet. Herbalists still recommend meadowsweet tea for fevers and aches and pains. Occasionally it is suggested as an eyewash, but no herb should ever be used for that purpose. If you are allergic to aspirin or salicylates, do not use meadowsweet.

❖ Melissa
See Balm.

❖ Mexican Wild Yam

See Wild Yam Root.

❖ Milk Thistle

Silybum marianum

A spiky plant with prickly leaves, milk thistle has small, hard seeds that were traditionally recommended for liver problems. The herb fell into disuse in modern times until the 1970s, when German scientists discovered that the seeds contained an antioxidant flavonoid they called silymarin. Their research bore out the traditional recommendation: silymarin does indeed have a valuable protective effect on the liver. In addition, silymarin has been found to stimulate the production of new liver cells. Because this could be helpful for people with hepatitis, cirrhosis, and other liver ailments, milk thistle is under active scientific investigation. In Germany, silymarin, usually as an injection, is used as a supportive treatment for liver disease. In the United States, silymarin is available only as a food supplement found in health food stores. Silymarin does not dissolve well in water, so milk thistle tea does not contain enough of the active ingredient to be helpful. Instead, herbal practitioners usually recommend taking several 200-milligram capsules a day. So far, there is no evidence that milk thistle capsules have any harmful effects. One word of caution: Be careful not to confuse milk thistle with another herb called blessed or holy thistle *(Cnicus benedictus)*.

❖ Mint

Mentha **spp.**

There are more than forty types of mint, but only a few are commonly used for their flavor and medicinal value. Spearmint and peppermint are the most popular, though pennyroyal and horehound (a member of the larger mint family) are also used. Peppermint contains the volatile oil menthol, which gives it most of its medicinal value. Spearmint, a closely related species, has no menthol and thus is used only as a flavoring.

The primary use for peppermint is as an aid to digestion. Sipping a hot cup or two of peppermint tea usually brings relief from indigestion, mild nausea, heartburn, and flatulence. Because it stimulates the stomach and relieves cramping, peppermint is an effective appetite stimulant. It also is often recommended for relieving mild menstrual cramps. Avoid giving peppermint to very young children. They can choke on the strong menthol flavor.

Menthol, an alcohol made from various mint oils, is sometimes used as a refrigerant, or cooling agent, for relieving sore muscles. In creams, ointment, or oil form, menthol is rubbed into the skin at the affected area as a counterirritant. It can be safely used three or four times a day.

Methyl salicylate, made from wintergreen (another distant member of the mint family), has the opposite effect from menthol. When ointments or creams containing methyl salicylate are rubbed into the skin, they induce a hot sensation. This counterirritation also helps relieve discomfort from aching muscles. Methyl salicylate can be safely used three or four times a day.

See also Horehound; Pennyroyal.

❖ Mistletoe

Viscum album or *Phoradendron* spp.

European mistletoe *(Viscum album)* is the red-berried plant under which you can be kissed at Christmas. American mistletoe (*Phoradendron* spp.) could be any one of at least four different species. European mistletoe has a long history as a magical and medicinal herb. It has been recommended as an herbal treatment for high blood pressure and anxiety, among other ailments. More recently, compounds found in European mistletoe have been used in Germany to treat tumors. For home use, however, European mistletoe is not advised. The berries are probably toxic, while little is known about the effects (particularly in the long run) of teas made from the leaves. The same is true of American mistletoe, the only difference being that these berries are definitely toxic. Avoid ingesting any sort of mistletoe.

❖ Mormon Tea
See Ephedra.

❖ Mugwort

Artemisia vulgaris

A close relative of the dangerous herb wormwood, mugwort is traditionally used as a bitter to stimulate the appetite and as treatment for menstrual discomfort. Mugwort can cause uterine contractions, among other undesirable side effects, and should not be taken internally.

In traditional Chinese medicine, mugwort is used to make

moxa sticks. These are burned at the end of acupuncture needles as part of the treatment known as moxibustion. Do not attempt to use moxa sticks yourself. If you are interested in moxibustion, see a trained acupuncturist.

See also Wormwood.

❖ Mullein

Vebascum spp.

A common roadside weed, mullein has been recommended as an herbal remedy for numerous ailments over the centuries, as well as for driving out evil spirits. Mullein's only real medicinal use, however, is as a moderately effective cough remedy, and it is often an ingredient included in herbal tea mixtures for coughs and colds. This herb has a high mucilage content, so a strong tea made from it can help soothe an irritated throat and help you cough up mucus. Herbalists tend to recommend mullein for hard, unproductive coughs.

❖ Mustard

Brassica spp.

Mustard, commonly used as a pungent table condiment, has uses outside the kitchen, chiefly as a heating agent. A good example is the traditional mustard plaster, used to relieve chest congestion from colds or flu. This is made by combining ground mustard seeds with water to form a thick paste and then spreading the paste on a piece of cloth. Next, the plaster is placed on the chest, with the cloth against the skin to prevent irritation, and left in place until it becomes uncomfortably warm for the patient. Do not leave the plaster in place for more than ten minutes, as skin blistering may occur. Do not use mustard plasters on babies, children, the elderly, or anyone with very sensitive skin.

Volatile mustard oil, which is distilled from ground mustard seeds, is sometimes used as a rubbing agent to relieve sore muscles. When rubbed into the affected area, the oil causes counterirritation and redness that, paradoxically, makes aching muscles feel better. Apply a few drops three or four times daily. Mustard oil is very pungent, but it is considered safe by the Food and Drug Administration. Do not, however, use volatile mustard oil near the eyes, face, or genitals. Because other rubbing agents, such as methyl salicylate (see the previous section on Mint), are equally effective and far less odorous, volatile mustard oil can't really be recommended.

❖ Myrrh

Commiphora myrrha

Since Biblical times, myrrh has been used as an essential ingredient in perfumes, as part of the embalming process, and as a drug to treat everything from indigestion to leprosy, but its effective medicinal uses today are restricted to mouthwashes. Myrrh is mildly astringent and antiseptic, so it is useful as a rinse for discomfort from mouth ulcers and sore gums and as a gargle for sore throats. It is also helpful in masking bad breath due to odorous foods such as garlic.

In its natural state, myrrh is a sap that dries into hard, rocklike crystals. Pieces of the hardened sap are used to make a tincture, which can be found in well-stocked health food stores. A few drops in a glass of water is all that is needed to make a homemade mouthwash.

❖ Nettle

See Stinging Nettle.

❖ Nightshade

See Deadly Nightshade.

❖ Nutmeg

Myristica fragrans

In the kitchen, nutmeg is a favorite spice for baking and seasoning. In herbal medicine, it is used chiefly for treating nausea and digestive upsets. Nutmeg is generally made into a tea or taken as capsules for this purpose. Nutmeg oil is also sometimes used for indigestion. Try putting a few drops onto a sugar cube or mixing them with honey. The oil can also be used for massage and to relieve arthritis pain. Rub a few drops into the skin at the site of the affected joint. A drop or two of nutmeg oil rubbed into the gums around an aching tooth can provide emergency relief. Use nutmeg with caution. Large doses (over 5 grams at a time) can cause convulsions and other serious side effects.

❖ Oat Bran

Avena sativa

Oat bran is the outer casing of the oat kernel; it is sold in bulk in health food stores as a coarse meal and is also available as a breakfast cereal. Two tablespoons of oat bran provide 1.8 grams of dietary fiber, 2.0 grams of protein, and 7.7 grams of carbohydrates. A daily serving of oats, either in the form of oatmeal or oat brain, could help lower your blood cholesterol levels because oat bran contains a lot of fiber and polyunsaturated fatty acids, which help bind up and remove LDL cholesterol from your system.

❖ Onions

Allium cepa

One of the world's oldest cultivated vegetables, onions (including leeks, shallots, scallions, and chives) are members of the lily family. They have been recommended as a healthful food for millennia. Indeed, the ancient Greek historian Herodotus advised the first Olympic athletes to eat onions to "lighten the balance of the blood." That recommendation is echoed by researchers today.

In addition to being rich in dietary fiber, vitamins, and minerals, onions are the richest dietary source of quercetin, a powerful, naturally occurring antioxidant compound. Preliminary studies suggest that quercetin may work to help prevent cancer cells and blood clots from forming, help inhibit allergic and inflammatory responses, and help stop infections. Onions also seem to have blood-thinning abilities because they contain adenosine, a naturally occurring chemical that has been shown to help lower LDL (bad) cholesterol in the blood and to lower blood pressure. Adenosine also plays an important role in inhibiting blood clots. The prostaglandins A1 and E, which play a role in naturally lowering blood pressure, have also been isolated in onions. It's no surprise, then, that cardiologists frequently advise heart patients to eat raw onions to help increase blood circulation, lower blood pressure, and reduce the chances of dangerous blood clots.

A major study in China, sponsored by the National Cancer Institute, showed that eating garlic and onions protects against stomach cancer. People in Shandong Province who ate 3 ounces of garlic and onions daily had far lower rates of stomach cancer than those who ate lesser amounts. In all probability, the sulfur compounds and quercetin in onions is responsible for the protective effect. The powerful anti-inflammatory effects of the quercetin in onions has also been shown to help asthma sufferers reduce the number and severity of their attacks.

❖ Oregon Grape

Mahonia aquifolium
See Barberry.

❖ Parsley

Petroselinum crispum
Parsley is a member of the umbelliferous vegetable family, which includes carrots, celery, dill, fennel, parsnips, and caraway. This vitamin-rich plant is a good source of dietary vitamin C. Natural medicine practitioners often recommend eating parsley for those taking the antibiotic drug tetracycline. They claim parsley helps offset the vitamin C depletion that may occur with this drug. Tea made from parsley is said to help relieve the symptoms of the common cold; some say it is also good for digestion and helps relieve stomach

cramps and flatulence. For a natural breath freshener, try chewing on fresh parsley sprigs.

Parsley also acts as a diuretic. Herbal practitioners sometimes recommend it to treat high blood pressure and edema from heart failure. These are serious conditions that should be treated by a physician. Do not attempt to treat high blood pressure or heart failure on your own with parsley.

❖ Passion Flower

Passiflora incarnata

The name of this showy South American flower refers to Christian religious symbolism, not passions of the more earthly sort. An extract made from the dried flowers was long used as a sedative for calming nerves and relieving insomnia, but since the late 1930s, it has not been popular in the United States. In 1978, the Food and Drug Administration removed passion flower from its list of herbs generally recognized as safe and effective, saying that it was ineffective as a sedative. However, passion flower remains popular in Europe, where it is an ingredient in many over-the-counter sleep aids and sedatives. If you suffer from insomnia, try having a cup of passion flower tea before bedtime. Steep 1 teaspoon of crushed leaves in 1 cup of boiling water for fifteen minutes. Strain before drinking. Passion flower tincture is sold in health food stores. For insomnia, try 1 teaspoon mixed with juice or any mild herbal tea.

❖ Pau d'Arco

Tabebuia spp.

People with cancer and other life-threatening illnesses are easy targets for unscrupulous sellers of herbs, and the marketing of pau d'arco is a good example. This herb, also known as lapacho or taheebo tea, is alleged to be a miraculous secret medicine known to the ancient Incas and is said to come from the bark of trees growing high in the Andes. In fact, it is very unclear where exactly the bark being sold as pau d'arco comes from, but it is probably from a lowland species found in Brazil.

When taken as a tea, pau d'arco supposedly cures cancer. As is often the case with miracle cures, however, the cancer-curing claim is based on dangerous extrapolation from animal studies. Lapachol, the active ingredient in pau d'arco, was found to have some effect against some very specific and rather rare types of animal cancer. In human trials, however, the side effects of doses large enough to be useful were so severe that the testing was stopped. If you have cancer or any other disease, you are very unlikely to benefit from pau d'arco, and you could make yourself sicker. Don't use it.

❖ Pennyroyal

Hedeoma pulgioides or *Mentha pulegium*

Pennyroyal is another member of the extended mint family. Its most popular use today is as an herbal insect repellent. A few drops of pennyroyal oil rubbed into the skin are said to repel mosquitos and other noxious insects and crushed pennyroyal leaves are sometimes used as a powder to keep fleas off pet dogs and cats. In addition, pennyroyal tea is sometimes recommended for stomach upsets. In all cases, however, pennyroyal should be used with extreme caution or not at all. Large amounts of pennyroyal oil can induce abortion, and even small amounts—less than 1 teaspoon—can be dangerous. Other, safer herbal remedies should be substituted for pennyroyal. Try citronella for repelling insects and peppermint for digestive upsets.

❖ Peppermint
See Mint.

❖ Periwinkle
See Tropical Periwinkle.

❖ Plantain/Plantago

Plantago spp.
Plantain is generally considered a lawn pest, but this ubiquitous weed has some very useful medicinal qualities. The fleshy leaves are an effective treatment for insect bites and stings. Crush the leaf and hold it against the bite. The crushed leaves are also effective for relieving the itching and oozing of poison ivy. When made into a tea, plantain leaves can be a useful home remedy for coughs. Steep 3 to 4 teaspoons in 1/2 cup of boiling water; take no more than 1 cup a day.

Plantain's greatest value comes from its numerous tiny seeds, particularly those from the species *Plantago psyllium*. Also called just psyllium (and sometimes called flea seeds), the seeds are a very effective bulking laxative. The seeds' husks are made up of soluble fiber, which means that they absorb water in the bowel and form a gel that adds bulk and softness to the stool. Over-the-counter bulk laxatives are made up largely of psyllium husks, often under the slightly misleading name of natural vegetable powder. If you wish to use psyllium as a laxative, don't try to harvest the seeds yourself. It's much easier and more effective to use a commercial brand.

❖ Pokeroot

Phytolacca americana
Pokeroot (also called pokeweed) was traditionally used by the Native Americans as a dye and as a general-purpose medicine. Although the blue-black berries of this roadside weed do make an effective dye or ink, they are toxic and should never be ingested or used for any medical purpose. In fact, no part of this plant, including the root, is safe. Don't use it.

❖ Pot Marigold
See Calendula.

❖ Propolis

A waxy brown substance produced by bees, propolis has mildly antibacterial and antifungal properties. It is available as a powder, extract, in cream, tablets, capsules, and as chips. A daily dose of propolis is said to stimulate the immune system. Proponents claim that propolis cures tuberculosis and ulcers. More realistically, propolis tincture applied externally may have some value as a treatment for minor bacterial and fungal infections of the skin, but it is unlikely to have much effect when taken internally for bacterial, fungal, or parasitic infections.

❖ Psyllium
See Plantain/Plantago.

❖ Purslane

Portulaca oleracea
Most people consider purslane, a sturdy green resembling clover, a weed. It's a weed with a nutritional wallop, however. Purslane is high in vitamins A, C, and E, magnesium, potassium, calcium, and omega-3 fatty acids. With a texture somewhat like sprouts and a nutty flavor, purslane can be added to salads, sautéed lightly and served as a side dish, or added to stews and soups for flavor and as a thickening agent.

❖ Raspberry Leaves

***Rubus* spp.**

The leaves of the red raspberry plant (and the botanically similar black raspberry) are often used to make a refreshing tea that can also be used as mouthwash and as a treatment for diarrhea. The high tannin content of raspberry leaf tea makes it quite astringent, which makes it an effective rinse for relieving mouth sores. It also works as a gargle for sore throats. The tannins in raspberry leaf tea make it moderately effective as a treatment for diarrhea, but the real benefit probably comes simply from the fluid the tea provides. Raspberry leaf tea is often recommended as a safe and enjoyable herbal drink during pregnancy. It has no caffeine, but it is high in tannin. To be on the safe side, don't drink more than 3 cups a day.

If you want to try raspberry leaf tea, be sure to purchase exactly that at the health food store. Don't purchase raspberry-flavored black tea or herbal mixes that contain only a small amount of raspberry leaves or raspberry flavoring. To make raspberry leaf tea, steep 1 to 2 teaspoons of the dried leaves in a cup of boiling water for ten to fifteen minutes (vary the amount of dried leaves and steeping time according to how much you like the strong tannin flavor).

❖ Red Clover

Trifolium pratense

Red clover was the main ingredient in the so-called Hoxey cure for cancer, a treatment that was offered from the 1930s through the 1950s at Hoxey's private clinics. This example of quack medicine proved completely ineffective, yet red clover is still sometimes touted as a cure for cancer and sexually transmitted diseases. Although red clover contains a range of active ingredients, including phenols, tannins, and tocopherol, that could possibly have antitumor action in a test tube, it has no therapeutic value for cancer or sexually transmitted diseases and should never be used to self-treat these serious conditions.

A more modest, if equally ineffective, use of red clover is as a tea for stimulating the appetite and for treating coughs.

❖ Rhubarb

Rheum spp.

The fibrous, pink to red stalks of rhubarb are thought to be native to northwest China and Tibet. The plant has been used there medicinally for over 2,000 years. The top, leafy portion of rhubarb contains a toxic amount of oxalate and should never be eaten. The stalk, which can range in color from pale green with pinkish overtones to a deep red, is extremely tart; generally, the redder the stalk, the less tart. Rhubarb stalks are high in calcium, but the mineral is in the form of calcium oxalate, which actually blocks the absorption of calcium by the body. The oxalate is also a hazard for people with kidney stones.

Rhubarb root (in powder or tincture form) is sometimes recommended as a laxative because it contains anthraquinones, which act as a powerful purgative. (Eating stalks from the supermarket or the garden has virtually no laxative effect.) Avoid using rhubarb root or any purgative laxatives. Their action is unpleasant to experience and could have serious side effects. If you are constipated, bulk-forming laxatives such as psyllium are a much gentler way to get relief.

❖ Rose

Rosa spp.

All parts of the rose blossom are used for various purposes in herbal medicine. The petals have a slightly astringent effect and are sometimes used in gargles and teas for sore throats, colds, and mouth irritations. More often, though, the petals are used to give color and fragrance to other preparations. An essential oil can be made from rose petals using a distillation process. In the French version, cabbage rose petals are distilled into a very expensive oil that is rumored to be an aphrodisiac. In the finer Bulgarian version, damask roses are used. Essential oil of rose is used primarily in perfumes; it is generally far too expensive and scarce to have any real use in herbal treatments. Rosewater, a by-product of the distillation process, is far less expensive and is sometimes used in herbal creams as a perfuming ingredient. Both rose oil and rosewater make nice additions to your bathwater for a soothing soak.

Rose hips, the bright red fruit left after the petals have fallen, have long been valued for their medicinal uses. They contain a fair amount of pectin, which makes them moderately useful as a natural laxative. They also have organic acids that make them a mild diuretic. Rose hips are an excellent source of natural vitamin C. The dried hips are often used in herbal teas to add vitamin C (and also vitamins A, B, E, and K) and flavor. Be wary when purchasing rose hips or rose hip tea at the health food store, however. While most fresh rose hips actually contain more vitamin C than an equivalent amount of orange, dried rose hips can vary considerably in their vitamin C content, depending on the type of rose and how the hips were collected and dried. Some rose hips sold in health food stores have virtually no vitamin C at all. Avoid buying rose hips that are very dry, faded, powdery, or smell musty. Likewise, many herbal tea mixtures that claim to have rose hips in them often contain only a small amount; these teas may also contain black tea and therefore will not be caffeine-free. To make a tea, steep 2 to

3 teaspoons chopped or crushed rose hips in 1 cup of boiling water for ten to fifteen minutes. Strain before drinking.

Natural vitamin C made from rose hips is considerably more expensive than synthetic vitamin C, but it isn't any better. Furthermore, many so-called natural vitamin C tablets contain only some vitamin C derived from rose hips. The rest is from synthetic ascorbic acid. Chemically speaking, the two are indistinguishable. In addition, powerful solvents are used to release vitamin C from rose hips.

❖ Rosemary

Rosemarinus officinalis
A common kitchen herb, rosemary had long been used in traditional herbal medicine for a range of ills. Today, rosemary's uses are far less broad. Try adding a handful of dried rosemary leaves to your bathwater, but not before bedtime. Rosemary is said to have an energizing effect. Oil of rosemary is sometimes used in creams, ointments, and liniments meant to relieve arthritis and muscle pain. In Europe, rosemary oil is used in ointments for varicose veins. Taken internally, it is used for indigestion (rosemary tea is also suggested). However, rosemary oil in large quantities can be very irritating to the kidneys and digestive tract. It could also bring on uterine contractions. Pregnant women should avoid rosemary oil and use the herb only for cooking.

❖ Royal Jelly

Royal jelly is a thick, whitish secretion made by worker bees to feed all bee larvae during their first three days of life. After that, if a bee larva continues to receive royal jelly, it grows into a queen bee, a fertile female who is considerably larger and lives longer than plain worker bees. One of the odder extrapolations of natural medicine is the belief that royal jelly has transformative effects on humans as well. Royal jelly has been said to help stop the aging process, improve sexual performance, restore hair loss, and cure anemia, arthritis, ulcers, and more. Although royal jelly does contain many of the B vitamins, including pantothenic acid, and also may have a mild antibiotic effect, it will certainly not stop the aging process, cure any disease, or perform any other magic feats.

❖ Rue

Ruta graveolens
At one time rue was widely used in European folk medicine, but this herb can be dangerous and should be avoided, especially by pregnant women. The volatile oils in rue can cause your skin to become photosensitive; it can also cause redness, blisters, and rashes. Taken internally, rue can cause intestinal pain, cramps, vomiting, confusion, and convulsions.

❖ Sabal
See Saw Palmetto.

❖ Sage

Salvia officinalis

Another member of the far-flung mint family, sage is a valuable culinary herb with a somewhat lemony, camphorlike flavor. According to ancient tradition, sage was said to cure most ills, improve the memory, and lengthen life spans. Today, sage does have value as a mouthwash or gargle for mouth irritations and sore throats. If you'd like to try it, make a tea using 1 to 2 teaspoons of dried sage; steep in 1 cup boiling water for ten minutes. Let cool and strain before using.

Sage is said to stop excessive perspiration. Little proof supports this claim, but an anhidrotic (antisweating) product made from sage is commercially available in Germany. Sage's volatile oil contains high concentrations of astringent compounds and also contains thujone, a dangerous poison that can cause convulsions and death. In culinary amounts, sage is perfectly safe to use. In larger medicinal amounts, however, it could be dangerous and should be avoided.

❖ St. John's Wort

Hypericum perforatum

Tea made from the leaves and flowers of St. John's wort, a perennial roadside weed with yellow flowers and a piney odor, is a popular European herbal remedy for depression. Drink no more than 3 cups of the tea a day. The antidepressant effect is not immediate. Herbalists generally suggest daily doses over several months. If you take St. John's wort for long periods, however, it could cause your skin to become sensitive to sunlight. If this occurs, stop using the herb until the photosensitivity goes away; take it less often or in smaller doses if you resume use.

Interestingly, St. John's wort contains hypericin, which has an effect similar to monoamine oxidase (MAO) inhibitors, a type of drug often prescribed for serious depression. People taking prescription MAO inhibitors are advised to avoid eating aged, fermented, and pickled foods, so it may be a good idea to avoid these foods, as well as any other drug, including nonprescription medications and amino acid supplements, if you are taking St. John's wort for long periods. MAO inhibitors are not recommended for people with high blood pressure and some other chronic problems because of negative side effects. St. John's wort in medicinal doses can cause nausea, stiff neck, and headache. If you are interested in using St. John's wort for depression, discuss doing so with your physician first.

St. John's wort tea is said to be very helpful for relieving premenstrual stress irritability. An infused oil made from St. John's wort petals is said to be helpful for arthritis and joint pain when rubbed into the skin at the affected area. Clinical trials of St. John's wort extract for treating AIDS symptoms have been inconclusive. It should be noted that in 1977 the Food and Drug Administration declared St. John's wort unsafe.

❖ Sanguinaria

See Bloodroot.

❖ Sarsaparilla

Smilax spp.

Sarsaparilla is made from the roots of any one of several climbing vines found in Central and South America. It has been used in the past as a blood purifier (a euphemism in this case for treating syphilis) and as a nonalcoholic beverage. Today, sarsaparilla is marketed to gullible athletes as a natural steroid that supposedly also contains testosterone. Of course, this is not true.

❖ Sassafras

Sassafras albidum
Until the 1960s, the pleasant aroma of sassafras bark was used to flavor root beer. The Food and Drug Administration, however, determined that the fragrance came from safrole oil, a carcinogenic substance, and banned the use of sassafras bark as a flavoring agent. It continues to be used in some ointments and liniments meant for external use only on aching muscles and joints. Sassafras is also said to help relieve itching from insect bites and poison ivy.

❖ Savory

Satureja spp.
Savory is a widely used culinary herb that is yet another member of the large mint family. It tastes a lot like a slightly sharper version of thyme. In the kitchen, savory is often added to beans to reduce gassiness. Try it to see if it works for you.

Medicinally, savory in the form of tea is sometimes suggested as a treatment for indigestion and flatulence. As such, it is mildly effective, but peppermint tea would be a better choice.

❖ Saw Palmetto

Serenoa serrulata or *Serenoa repens*

Saw palmetto, also called sabal, has shown some promise for the treatment of benign prostatic hyperplasia (BPH). Over-the-counter preparations containing an extract of saw palmetto are used to treat mild BPH symptoms in Canada and Germany. In the United States, however, the Food and Drug Administration does not allow nonprescription remedies containing saw palmetto to be sold as treatments for BPH. It is possible to purchase saw palmetto extract in an alcohol base in the U.S. in health food stores. The suggested daily dose is usually 30 to 60 drops mixed with liquid. (Using the plant parts as a tea or decoction is unlikely to be effective because the active ingredient is not water soluble.) If you have prostate disease of any sort, or if you are experiencing difficulty in urinating for any reason, discuss using saw palmetto with your physician before you try it.

❖ Schisandra

Schisandra chinensis

In traditional Chinese herbal medicine, berries from the schisandra tree (also called wu wei zi) are used as a liver treatment (especially for hepatitis) and overall tonic. Modern-day herbalists tout schisandra as an adaptogen that supposedly helps stimulate your immune system and increase your energy levels. Schisandra has been studied for its beneficial effects on the liver, but the results are far from definitive. In one animal study, the amount needed to protect the liver against harmful substances was in itself toxic to the liver. Other studies have failed to prove that schisandra has any sort of stimulating effect on the body.

❖ Seaweed

Laminaria **spp.,** *Macrocystis* **spp.,** *Nereocystis*
spp., *Fucus vesiculosus,* **others**

Seaweed (also called sea vegetable) is used in many Asian
cuisines, notably Japanese, and its many health benefits may
encourage a greater consumption throughout the rest of the
world. A wide variety of seaweeds are used for culinary purposes, and each has its own unique taste and nutritional
composition. Kelp (also called bladderwrack) is one of the
most familiar. It has no fat, no cholesterol, is extremely low
in calories, and provides generous amounts of folate, iodine
(essential for your thyroid gland, but a possible cause of
acne flare-ups in some people), magnesium, and, in smaller
amounts, calcium and iron. Fresh kelp can be added to soup
stocks for color and flavor; dried kelp (known as kombu) is
used to wrap sushi and can be brewed as a tea. Other forms
of edible seaweed include carrageenan (also called Irish
moss), which is thought to prevent ulcers and blood clots;
laminaria, which may help prevent high blood pressure and
hardening of the arteries; hijiki or hiziki, a good source of
dietary fiber, potassium, magnesium, riboflavin, and calcium; wakame, whose nutrient breakdown is similar to hijiki; and arame, which provides generous amounts of fiber,
vitamin A, zinc, and calcium. Dulse and laver, North Atlantic seaweeds, are similar in nutritional content to hijiki.

  Eating seaweed is sometimes suggested as a means of
protecting your body against harmful heavy metal accumulation. The theory behind this is that radiation, including
strontium 90, and toxic heavy metals, such as cadmium and
plutonium, accumulate in your bones as a result of daily exposure to a polluted world; eventually, the accumulation can
cause cancers such as leukemia or Hodgkin's disease. The
sodium alginate in the seaweed helps prevent the absorption
of additional radiation and heavy metals, although it doesn't
do anything for any accumulation you might already have. If
you are routinely exposed to radiation or heavy metals as

part of your work, you might consider taking kelp supplements on a regular basis as a preventive measure. Otherwise, there is little evidence that seaweed can prevent cancer. Despite claims, seaweed will not cure or prevent heart disease, arthritis, liver problems, sexually transmitted diseases, infections, or high blood pressure.

Iodine is routinely added to table salt, so it is very unlikely that anyone in North America would ever have thyroid trouble (causing weight gain) as a result of an iodine deficiency. If your thyroid function is normal, merely adding seaweed to your diet will not make you lose weight.

❖ Senega Snakeroot

Polygala senega
Senega snakeroot is the root of a plant native to eastern North America. Originally, it was used by the Native Americans (hence the name) as a cure for snakebite (ineffective), and as a treatment for colds and coughs. Today, herbalists suggest Senega snakeroot as an asthma and bronchitis remedy; it is also an ingredient in many over-the-counter European cough medicines. In very small amounts, Senega snakeroot is mildly effective as an expectorant for coughs, but even fairly small doses can cause nausea and vomiting. In general, there is no reason to use this herb for coughs when there are more effective alternatives that are far less likely to have unpleasant side effects. If you have asthma or bronchitis, discuss any herbal remedies with your doctor before you try them.

❖ Senna

Cassia spp.

Senna, also known as cassia, is a very potent laxative that should be used with great caution. In addition to its purgative effects and awful taste, senna causes unpleasant griping and nausea; the effects can continue for several hours or longer and could cause dangerous dehydration. Senna is an ingredient in a number of nonprescription laxatives, but if you are constipated, bulk-forming laxatives such as psyllium are a much gentler way to get relief. In general, don't use senna unless your physician recommends it.

❖ Shepherd's Purse

Capsella bursa-pastoris

A common roadside weed, shepherd's purse gets its name from its small, heart-shaped seed pods. The pods are filled with many tiny seeds, suggesting the purse of someone who is very poorly paid. Musings on shepherds' wages aside, this herb has little to recommend it. Although it is sometimes recommended by herbalists for controlling heavy menstrual bleeding and for stopping bleeding from nosebleeds, cuts, and wounds, it is basically ineffective. Applying shepherd's purse to an open wound could cause infection. Don't do it. This herb does contain compounds that can cause uterine contractions. Pregnant women should avoid shepherd's purse.

❖ Shiitake

Lentinus edodes

Shiitake mushrooms, a popular Japanese species, contain a substance called lentinan, which the Japanese use as a treatment for cancer. Recent studies suggest that lentinan stimulates the immune system, which may help the body fight off cancer and viral infections such as AIDS and flu. Promising as this research is, you won't get the beneficial effects simply by eating lots of these mushrooms. Laboratory experiments use mushroom extracts. On a more practical note, eating 3 ounces of shiitake mushrooms a day could have a slight beneficial effect on your blood cholesterol level. Shiitake mushrooms are now commercially cultivated in the United States and are readily available in the produce section.

❖ Siberian Ginseng

Eleutherococcus senticosus

Calling this root Siberian ginseng is very misleading, because it is not at all related to the ginseng family. It should really be known by its other name, eleuthero, but most herbal practitioners and health food stores insist on Siberian ginseng. This herb, whatever you choose to call it, is widely used in traditional Chinese herbal medicine as a general tonic. It is said to have the same mildly stimulating effect as ginseng and to be a good alternative for those who find ginseng too strong or too expensive. However, be very cautious about purchasing Siberian ginseng. Mislabeling and poor quality control are widespread. Analyses of capsules said to contain Siberian ginseng have shown that they often contain a completely different herb or have caffeine or other adulterants added to them. Given the possible uncertainties, this is an herb to avoid.

See also Ginseng.

❖ Skullcap

Scutellaria spp.

Skullcap is one of those herbs that inexplicably continue to be recommended, despite a complete lack of effectiveness. Herbalists suggest using the aerial parts in a tea for insomnia, nerves, anxiety, and premenstrual stress. The root, sometimes called huang chin, is used in traditional Chinese herbal medicine as a tonic for "hot" conditions. Though skullcap offers no observable benefits, in large amounts it could cause liver damage. In addition, the herb sold as skullcap is often adulterated with or replaced by another herb, germander. Avoid this herb.

❖ Slippery Elm

Ulmus fulva or Ulmus rubra

The inner bark of the elm tree contains large amounts of mucilage. When ground into a fine powder and mixed with water, the inner bark forms a slippery gel that can have a soothing effect on sore throats and the digestive tract. In fact, slippery elm is an ingredient in some throat lozenges sold in pharmacies and health food stores. As a poultice, slippery elm is sometimes used to treat skin irritations and to cover minor wounds.

Because North America is no longer covered with great forests of elms (they were killed off by Dutch elm disease in the late 1800s and early 1900s), slippery elm is sometimes hard to find. To make it into a decoction for sore throats, mix 1 or 2 teaspoons with a little cold water in a small saucepan to form a smooth paste. Add 1 cup of water and bring to a boil. Simmer for fifteen minutes, let cool to room temperature, and drink. Take no more than 3 cups a day. To make a poultice, make a thick paste of powdered bark and water; spread it on the affected area, and let it dry.

❖ Snakeroot
See Senega Snakeroot.

❖ Spirulina

Spirulina spp.
One of the primitive blue green algae that are among the earliest forms of life on earth, spirulina is marketed today as a natural source of chlorophyll, amino acids, vitamins, and minerals—and as a way to lose weight quickly without dieting. One 500-milligram spirulina tablet with each meal will supposedly control your appetite, suppress hunger pangs, and help you eat less. The scientific basis for the efficacy of spirulina is said to be the amino acid L-phenylalanine, which is believed to have an influence on the brain's appetite control center. This claim was carefully reviewed by the Food and Drug Administration in 1979 and found to be baseless.

❖ Squaw Tea

See Ephedra.

❖ Stinging Nettle

Urtica dioica

The tiny hairs that cover the leaves of the stinging nettle plant produce pain and itching when they come in contact with your skin. Herbalists, reasoning perhaps that a plant with such a kick just has to be good for you, recommend stinging nettle to stimulate the immune system and as a treatment for a variety of other conditions, including arthritis, gout, and sciatica. It is ineffective for these purposes, although the fresh leaves are a moderately good source of vitamin C. Stinging nettle's one possible medicinal use is as a diuretic. German physicians sometimes prescribe nettle juice for high blood pressure or heart failure. Do not try stinging nettle for these serious conditions without discussing it with your physician first.

❖ Suma

Pfaffia paniculata

Sometimes called Brazilian ginseng, suma is a plant from South America that has recently become popular as an immune system booster and healing tonic. It contains pfaffic acid, which some Japanese researchers claim may inhibit the growth of cancer cells. Proponents of suma claim that it has been used for centuries in Brazil as a folk remedy for a variety of ailments. There is no evidence that this is true and neither is there any evidence that using suma is safe or effective. This is another herb to avoid.

❖ Tansy

Tanacetum vulgare

Strong-tasting tansy tea was once widely used in folk medicine, especially for skin problems and intestinal parasites. However, tansy contains thujone, the same dangerous volatile oil found in wormwood. Thujone can cause convulsions, hallucinations, and psychosis. Small amounts of tansy are safe when used for culinary purposes, but never use tansy medicinally.

❖ Tea

Camellia sinensis

A nice cup of tea may not only cheer you up, it may also help prevent cancer, heart attacks, strokes, ulcers, osteoporosis, and even tooth decay. Numerous studies have documented the value of the various compounds found in green, oolong, and black tea.

All of these teas are made from the leaves of *Camellia sinensis,* a flowering evergreen plant native to parts of India and China. Today, most tea is grown on plantations in India, Sri Lanka, Indonesia, and China. The different types of tea are the result of different ways of handling the fresh leaves.

Green tea, often served in Asian restaurants, is made from leaves that have been steamed, rolled, and then heated. The final product is high in tannin, with a delicate perfume, a mild flavor, and a light color when brewed. Commercially, green tea is also sometimes called gunpowder tea. Oolong tea is made by letting the fresh leaves wilt, rather than steaming them. The leaves are then rolled and left to ferment naturally for a time (for this reason, oolong tea is also sometimes called semifermented tea). The leaves are then heated to stop the fermentation process. Oolong tea is darker and more flavorful than green tea; it has less tannin and less aroma. Black tea (the familiar tea found in commercial tea bags) is made much like oolong tea, but the fermentation process is allowed to proceed longer. The flavor produced is strong and full. Black tea is also sometimes called Pekoe or Orange Pekoe tea. Flavorings are sometimes added to black tea; for example, Earl Grey is flavored with oil of bergamot, a citrus fruit. All of these teas contain caffeine, but a cup of brewed tea has far less caffeine than an equivalent cup of brewed coffee. In general, green tea has less caffeine than black or oolong tea.

Tea contains numerous substances that can contribute to good health. Catechins, a chemical compound found in tea, seem to help lower blood cholesterol levels and prevent atherosclerosis, or the buildup of dangerous plaque in your arteries. Catechins may also help protect you against cancer. A study in Japan suggests that people who drink a lot of green tea are less likely to get stomach cancer. Green tea has the most catechins and thus the most potent anticancer effect. Because catechins are reduced by the fermenting process, oolong and black teas have less. Tea also contains antioxidant vitamin C and the minerals boron and manganese (vital for strong bones and preventing osteoporosis). If you drink tea after eating, you could reduce your incidence of cavities, since tea contains antibiotic substances that can kill the germs that cause tooth decay.

❖ Tea Tree Oil

Melaleuca alternifolia

Tea tree oil has nothing to do with tea. Rather, it is made from the leaves of an Australian tree of the myrtle family. Tea tree oil has long had a folk reputation in Australia as an effective treatment for minor skin irritations, cuts, scrapes, and burns. It is also said to have antifungal action and be useful for treating athlete's foot. Studies indicate that this aromatic, amber-colored oil may indeed be a useful natural remedy. Try it as an alternative to nonprescription antibiotic or cortisone ointments, or instead of benzoyl peroxide for treating acne. Tea tree oil is now readily available in health food stores.

❖ Thyme

Thymus vulgaris

Thyme is a very popular cooking herb and also has a long history of medicinal use. Tea made from thyme leaves is a traditional treatment for stomach upsets, colds, coughs (thyme is a flavoring ingredient in some commercial cough remedies), chest congestion, and menstrual cramps. Herbalists usually recommend drinking no more than 3 cups a day of thyme tea.

Thyme gets its characteristic aroma and taste from thymol, an oil that has useful antiseptic qualities. Thyme oil was widely used as an antiseptic until well into this century. In fact, the distinctive taste of thymol is recognizable in some commercial mouthwashes said to kill the germs that cause bad breath. Thyme oil is sometimes recommended as a chest rub, as an ointment for skin irritations and insect bites, and as a massage oil. However, thyme oil can cause irritation of the skin and mucus membranes and could cause uterine contractions in pregnant women. Taken internally, even a few spoonfuls could be toxic. While thyme tea in moderation is generally safe, avoid using thyme oil.

❖ Tropical Periwinkle

Catharanthus rosens
Many people are alive today because of two drugs derived from tropical periwinkle: vinblastine and vincristine. These powerful drugs are used to cure leukemia, Hodgkin's disease, breast cancer, and lymphoma. Simply because a valuable medicine is made from a plant, however, does not mean you can use it to treat yourself or anyone else. Drugs made from tropical periwinkle have significant side effects, and overdoses can be life-threatening. Even a simple tea made from the leaves or flowers could be very dangerous.

Tropical periwinkle is native to Madagascar, but today it is often grown elsewhere in humid, hot climates as an ornamental. Use it only for that purpose.

❖ Turmeric

Curcuma longa
For centuries, Ayurvedic practitioners in India have used powdered turmeric root as a treatment for liver and gallbladder problems, as an aid to digestion, and as treatment for a wide range of other problems. Likewise, traditional Chinese herbalists have long recommended turmeric for liver ail-

ments and menstrual difficulties. To Americans, turmeric is known chiefly for its vivid yellow color (used in commercial mustard) and for its culinary use as an ingredient in curries.

Should turmeric be considered a valuable healing herb or just a cooking spice? Probably the latter—and even then, some caution is required. Turmeric can be of some help as a digestive aid because it stimulates your gallbladder to release bile. Some studies suggest that turmeric contains beneficial anticlotting compounds similar to those found in ginger. Some animal studies suggest that turmeric could help protect your liver and relieve arthritis symptoms. There is some evidence, however, that turmeric—even the amounts found in curry powder—could actually worsen gallstones or a blocked bile duct. If you have gallbladder trouble, avoid turmeric. If you have a clotting disorder, liver disease, or arthritis, discuss turmeric with your doctor before you try it.

❖ Uva Ursi

Arctostaphylos uva-ursi

Uva ursi (also called bearberry) is a traditional herbal treatment for urinary tract infections. The leaves of this plant have an antiseptic and diuretic effect that can be helpful for bladder problems. Because uva ursi also contains large amounts of tannins, which can cause stomach upsets, herbalists usually recommend making a cold infusion from the leaves. For the best results, soak 1/2 cup of uva ursi leaves in 2 quarts of cold water for twelve to twenty-four hours. Strain before using. The usual dose is 1 cup of the tea up to six times a day. In large doses, uva ursi can give the urine a harmless dark green color.

Uva ursi works best if your urine is alkaline. If you are using it for a bladder complaint, avoid acid-rich foods such as citrus juices; don't take supplemental vitamin C. Uva ursi is readily available in health food stores. It is often the chief ingredient in tea mixtures for the bladder and kidneys. It is also often a main ingredient in weight-loss teas that seem to work because of their diuretic effect. Do not use uva ursi or other diuretics to lose weight. Dehydration and other serious problems could result.

❖ Valerian

Valeriana officinalis

Valerian root is an ancient and effective remedy for insomnia. This safe natural tranquilizer is often taken as a tea before bedtime. To make it, steep 2 teaspoons of dried valerian root in 1 cup of boiling water for fifteen minutes. To disguise the tea's pungent taste, try adding a few drops of peppermint oil and a spoonful of honey. If you prefer, try a few drops of valerian root tincture (available at health food stores).

Valerian root is an ingredient in many over-the-counter sleep aids sold in Europe, where it is widely recommended by physicians. Although this is a safe herb with few side effects, don't use it with any other sort of sedative drug, prescription or nonprescription. Don't use it continually for more than a week. In large doses, valerian can lower your blood pressure. Don't use valerian if you take medication for high blood pressure.

Despite the similarity in their names and uses, valerian has no relation to the prescription drug Valium (diazepam).

❖ Vervain

Verbena officinalis

As a medicinal herb, vervain has been popular with everyone from the ancient Egyptians to the Druids of northern
Europe, to say nothing of medieval herbalists. Its uses were
just as widespread. Vervain was recommended for acne,
menstrual discomfort, "pain in the secret parts," toothache,
insomnia, and liver problems. There is no evidence that vervain affects any of these conditions, but many people swear
that a cup or two of strong vervain tea or a teaspoon of vervain tincture relieves minor aches and pains and headaches.
Vervain is also one of the herbs used in the Bach flower
remedies. Vervain tea has a mildly bitter taste that many
people find refreshing and relaxing.

❖ Virginia Snakeroot

Aristolochia serpentaria

It's easy to confuse the many medicinal herbs that have the
word snakeroot as part of their names. However, take care
not to confuse Virginia snakeroot with anything else. It's a
dangerous herb that should never be used. If you have the
slightest doubt as to what kind of snakeroot is being offered,
don't use it.

See also Senega Snakeroot.

❖ Vitex

Verbenaceae spp.

Vitex, also called chaste tree, is popular in Europe as an herbal treatment for PMS, menstrual problems, and menopause symptoms. The berry of this small shrub contains substances that inhibit the production of the hormone prolactin. Since women who suffer from amenorrhea (lack of periods) sometimes have elevated prolactin levels, it is possible that vitex works by lowering prolactin levels. The active ingredients in vitex are still poorly understood, however, and this herb should be used with caution. Do not use vitex to treat fibroid tumors. If you wish to use vitex to treat any other problem, discuss it with your doctor first.

❖ Wahoo

Euonymus atropurpureus

Wahoo is definitive proof that not every herb used by the Native Americans is safe. All parts of this plant, including the bark, leaves, and berries, are dangerously toxic. Wahoo is unsafe and should not be used for any purpose.

❖ Wheat Bran

A kernel or berry of wheat is the seed of the wheat plant. It consists of the bran (the outer hull of the kernel), the endosperm (the interior of the kernel), and the germ (the sprouting section at the base of the endosperm). Wheat kernels are ground to make flour. If the bran is left on the kernel before grinding, the result is whole wheat flour. If the bran is removed, the result is white flour.

Wheat bran (also sometimes called miller's bran) is sold separately in health food stores. It can vary in color from tan to dark red brown. Depending on the method of milling, the consistency can range from powdery to flaky. It's primary use is as a supplement to provide dietary fiber, but wheat bran is also a good source of B vitamins and copper. Some evidence suggests that eating wheat bran can reduce a woman's risk of breast cancer by lowering the levels of estrogen in the blood. Wheat bran also contains phytate, a substance that has been shown to prevent color cancer in animals—and possibly in humans as well.

❖ Wheat Germ

The germ in wheat germ isn't a bacteria. Rather, it is the tiny portion of a wheat kernel that sprouts when the seed is planted. Because it is high in oil, the germ is often removed from the kernel when milling wheat for flour; otherwise, the flour would become rancid if not used quickly. Wheat germ is slightly crunchy and has a delicious, slightly nutty flavor that is packed with nutrition. A quarter cup of wheat germ has 8.3 grams of high-quality protein, 3.7 grams of insoluble dietary fiber, and is an excellent source of vitamin E, folic acid, riboflavin, niacin, zinc, thiamine, iron, magnesium, and potassium.

As health foods go, wheat germ is unusually palatable. It can be added to casseroles, baked goods, and pancakes or sprinkled on oatmeal, yogurt, fruit, or anything else. The high fat content in wheat germ, however, can cause it to

spoil quickly. Store it in a sealed container in the refrigerator
for up to six months.

❖ White Oak Bark

Quercus alba

The inner bark of the white oak contains large amounts of
tannins. When the dried bark is powdered and made into a
decoction, it is a useful (but very bitter-tasting) rinse for
minor mouth irritations. It can also be applied to the skin to
relieve minor irritations such as poison ivy and insect bites.
To make a white oak bark decoction, use 1 teaspoon ground
bark for each cup of boiling water. Let steep for fifteen minutes and strain before using.

❖ White Willow Bark

Salix alba

The dried inner bark of the white willow has been used over
the centuries by many cultures as a treatment for fever, pain,
and inflammation. The active ingredient in white willow
bark is salicin. When salicin is synthesized in the laboratory,
it is known as acetylsalicylic acid, or, more familiarly, aspirin. The problem with white willow bark is that it doesn't
contain very much salicin, and what there is, is mixed with
very bitter-tasting tannins. Although white willow bark tea
is often recommended as a natural pain reliever, particularly
for the discomfort of arthritis, you would have to drink very
large amounts—a minimum of several strong cups—and

wait a couple of hours to get the same relief as one aspirin tablet. Some people object to aspirin because it upsets their stomach. White willow bark is so high in tannins, however, that it is even more likely to cause stomach upset, whether taken as a tea or as a tincture or in capsules containing powdered bark. Since the active ingredient in both white willow bark and aspirin is essentially identical, it is far cheaper, easier, and more effective to take aspirin tablets to relieve minor muscle and joint pain.

❖ Wild Yam Root

Dioscorea spp.

Wild yam root (also called Mexican wild yam) contains compounds that were used in early efforts to synthesize oral contraceptives and sex hormones. Unfortunately, some irresponsible herbalists today recommend an extract of the root as a contraceptive and for other medicinal purposes. Do not use wild yam root for any purpose. If you wish to use an oral contraceptive, discuss it with your doctor.

❖ Wintergreen

See Mint.

❖ Witch Hazel

Hamamelis virginiana

Witch hazel extract is a widely used preparation available in any drugstore, yet when most people use it, they don't realize that it is an herbal remedy. In fact, witch hazel was used for its astringent qualities by the Native Americans long before settlers arrived in North America. Witch hazel soon became popular with the colonists as a treatment for skin problems and hemorrhoids, which remain the two primary uses of witch hazel today.

An extract made from witch hazel leaves and bark is an astringent that is quite high in tannins. When applied to inflamed skin or hemorrhoids, witch hazel reduces swelling and relieves pain; it can also help relieve discomfort from varicose veins when applied to the skin at the site of the affected area. Unfortunately, the witch hazel commonly sold in pharmacies is made using a distillation process that produces an alcoholic extract with very little tannin. If distilled witch hazel extract has any effect at all, it is as a result of the alcohol.

If you wish to use witch hazel as an aftershave lotion or as a treatment for minor skin problems such as poison ivy, sunburn, or insect bites, or if you wish to use it for varicose veins or hemorrhoids, be sure to purchase nondistilled witch hazel extract. If you can't find it at your pharmacy, check your health food store.

❖ Wood Betony

See Betony.

❖ Wormwood

Artemisia absinthium

In the late 1800s and early 1900s, wormwood was used to give absinthe, a popular and potent alcoholic beverage, its bitter flavor—and also its danger. Wormwood contains thujone, a powerful oil that can cause convulsions, hallucinations, and death. Habitual and even occasional absinthe drinkers sometimes became seriously ill or psychotic; some died. After much public outcry, absinthe was banned in most countries by 1915.

Herbalists today still sometimes recommend wormwood to treat intestinal parasites, as an appetite stimulant, for menstrual discomfort, and for a range of other ailments. Wormwood is far too risky for home use, however, and should be avoided.

See also Mugwort.

❖ Yarrow

Achillea millefolium

Yarrow is closely related to chamomile and is used for many of the same purposes. It is somewhat less effective than chamomile for relieving indigestion, although many say it is slightly more effective for relieving menstrual discomfort.

If you are allergic to ragweed, avoid yarrow. It's likely that you are allergic to it as well.

See also Chamomile.

❖ Yellow Dock

Rumex crispus

Yellow dock (sometimes called dock) has traditionally been recommended for liver ailments and as a tonic and blood purifier. The root of this perennial herb does have a laxative effect similar to that of rhubarb, but otherwise it has no value. Do not use yellow dock as a laxative, as an herbal remedy, or for any other purpose.

Yellow dock leaves are sometimes eaten as a vegetable, but be careful. The leaves are high in vitamin C, but they also contain large amounts of oxalic acid. Even if you don't have gout (which is made worse by this chemical), the oxalic acid level is so high that it could cause digestive discomfort.

❖ Yerba Maté
See Maté.

❖ Yohimbe

Pausinystalia yohimba

A vast number of herbs and other substances are said to help impotence. Most of these claims are nonsense, but yohimbe is one herb that may actually work. The bark of a tree found in west Africa, yohimbe contains alkaloids that do seem to improve erectile function in some men. Yohimbe is widely available in Germany as a prescription drug and in a stunning range of allegedly aphrodisiac potions sold over the counter. It is approved for use in the United States only as a prescription drug. This is because yohimbe can have serious side effects, including anxiety, diabetes, liver disease, or kidney disease. The Food and Drug Administration considers yohimbe to be unsafe and ineffective in nonprescription formulations and has banned it from over-the-counter sales.

❖ Yucca

Yucca spp.

The Native Americans of the Southwest prized the yucca plant for its fibrous qualities. They used the plant to make sandals, baskets, cords, and the like, but they don't seem to have used it for any medicinal purpose. In the 1970s, however, claims for yucca extract as a miracle treatment for arthritis began to be heard. As is usual in such cases, the miraculous claims did not hold up to examination. Yucca is not an effective treatment for arthritis.

An expert authority on nutrition, **Dr. David Kessler** has had an active New York practice, specializing in family medicine, for over twenty years. Dr. Kessler received his M.D. from Albany Medical College. In addition, he was recently named a diplomate of the National Board of Examiners, and is a diplomate of the American Board of Family Practice.

Sheila Buff is a professional medical writer and the author of over twenty books to date, including *All About Nonprescription Drugs and Vitamins*. In addition, she is the Managing Director of Ibid. Editorial Services.

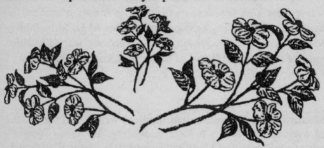